CERVICAL DYSPLASIA & PROSTATE CANCER: HPV, A HIDDEN LINK?

Cervical Dysplasia & Prostate Cancer HPV, A Hidden Link?

The Diagnosis & Treatment Of Cervical Intraepithelial Neoplasia & Prostate Problems Based On Traditional Chinese Medical Theory & A Rational, Multimodal Approach To Therapy Utilizing A Combination Of TCM, Western Naturopathy & Clinical Ecology

by

Bob Flaws

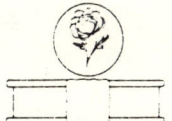

Blue Poppy Press

Published by:

BLUE POPPY PRESS
1775 LINDEN AVE.
BOULDER, CO 80304

FIRST EDITION
NOVEMBER 1990

ISBN 0-936185-19-8

COPYRIGHT © BLUE POPPY PRESS

All rights reserved. No part of this book may be reproduced, stored in a retrieval system, or transcribed in any form or by any means, electronic, mechanical, photocopy, recording, or any other means, without the prior written permission of the publisher.

Printed at Westview Press, Boulder, CO
Cover printed at D & K Printing, Boulder, CO

This book is printed on archive quality, acid free, recycled paper.

ACKNOWLEDGEMENTS

Because this book is about the combination of modern Western medicine and Traditional Chinese Medicine (TCM) and because I am only trained as a professional practitioner of TCM, I have had to depend upon the knowledge, advice, and opinions of others more specifically trained in Western biomedical science. Therefore, thanks are due to Kathleen Belko, DC, Dipl. Ac., for elucidation of the embryological relationships between the cervix and prostate; to Jody Shevins, ND, for sharing of information on Western naturopathic protocols for cervical dysplasia; to Johanna Riley, ND, for information on modern homeopathy; to Patrick Gourley, RN, for furnishing research materials on HPV; to Jack Finch, MS, of the Cancer Control Registry, Colorado Department of Health, for furnishing me with statistical information on both cervical and prostate cancers; to Edward Di Antoni also of the Cancer Control Section, Colorado Department of Health for information on CIN screening and follow-up; to Carol Rupp and Kristy Hendricks of Metagenics West, Denver, for supplying me with research materials on orthomolecular medicinals and supporting me in my attempts at describing these as TCM medicinals; to Rachel Fresco at K'an Herbs for supplying me with research materials on Bioradiance and to Lila Berkheim at Apex Energetics who kindly supplied me with information and materials for the biokinesiological *cum* nosode testing for HPV. I must also thank William C. Blake, archivist and conservator at the Lloyd Museum in Cincinnati for helping me research Western herbs for this book. In addition, Charles Chace, Dipl.Ac., and Zhang Ting-liang, Dipl.Ac., helped with translating Qin Bo-wei's essay on the *Ming Men* which appears in Appendix II.

Beyond these professional acknowledgements, I must always and ever thank my wife, Honora Lee Wolfe, for doing so much of the word processing, design, and layout of this and all my books. In particular, I am grateful for her patience in living with me as I wrestled with some of the conceptual difficulties in writing this book.

FOREWORD

As a practitioner of Traditional Chinese Medicine (TCM) specializing in gynecology, I have noticed an alarming increase in cervical dysplasia amongst my patients. Although I have treated cervical dysplasia on an occasional basis the entire 10 years I have been in practice, in the last 2 years I have seen more cases than the previous 8 together. This increase has caused me a great deal of thought on the subject of dysplasia and its TCM treatment.

During roughly the same 2 years, one close family member and one family friend have had to be treated surgically for benign prostatic hypertrophy and prostate cancer. This, likewise, has caused me considerable thought on the cause and treatment of prostate problems, stimulated further by the fact that, as a man in my mid-40s, I myself am entering a phase of life during which I am at jeopardy for prostate problems.

Curiously, in my research and thought on these two seemingly disparate diseases, I have uncovered a possible link suggesting that they may, in fact, be the same disease process taking but a different form because of differences in sexual anatomy. This book is the presentation and explication of this surmised link between cervical dysplasia in women and prostate problems in men.

Because I am a TCM gynecologist, my expertise in treating cervical dysplasia, based on my greater clinical experience with that disease, is disproportionately evident. In this book, TCM clinicians will find, I think, a wealth of practical information on the treatment and management of this problem. In these pages, I have given empirically tested protocols for the remedial treatment of cervical dysplasia and preventive regimes for barring its recurrence. *In my 10 years of practice, no woman who has followed these protocols has failed to get a negative Pap smear.*

As for prostate problems, my emphasis in this book is on early prevention. It is my feeling that, through diet, orthomolecular, herbal, homeopathic, and acupuncture therapies, men at risk for prostate problems can do a great deal to reduce the likelihood of prostate disease. Although my suggestions have yet to be validated by clinical experience, TCM theory on this matter seems clear enough to support the validity of my approach. Because of the nature of prostate problems, it will take many years before I or anyone else will know for sure how effective the preventive regimes I suggest actually are.

In addition to providing my fellow clinicians with protocols for these problems, this book also attempts to elucidate and clarify the treatment of chronic viral infections in general. Based on the information contained herein, practitioners should glean much useful insight into the treatment and management of Epstein-Barr virus (EBV), herpes simplex II (HSV II or herpes genitalia), cytomegalovirus (CMV), and even human immune-deficiency virus (HIV, aka AIDS). These are some of the most important diseases modern clinicians are faced with treating today.

Traditional Chinese Medicine has a lot to say about and a lot of useful treatment to offer for these and other chronic viral infections. Its theory is wise enough to allow a great deal of insight into the mechanisms of these diseases. Likewise, its theory is also broad enough to allow the incorporation of new therapies which, when used in tandem with TCM's older, more standard therapies, achieve even better, more satisfactory results.

It is no mere coincidence that the theories most helpful in understanding the cause and treatment of chronic viral infection in general and cervical dysplasia and prostate problems in particular are derived from Qing Dysnaty *Wen Bing Xue* or Warm Disease theory. *Wen Bing Xue* was developed in response to the epidemic, febrile diseases which became prevalent in the 17th, 18th, and 19th Centuries. Likewise, it is further development of this same line of reasoning which holds promise of providing the theoretical basis for the treatment of viral diseases of the 20th and 21st Centuries.

This clearly shows that TCM is a still evolving medicine and not some medical anachronism or *fait accompli* per chance surviving into the modern world. In the Native American tradition, it is believed that the treatment of any disease (or the solution of any problem, for that matter) lies within the patient's Medicine Wheel. This means that a cure or solution is within the patient's immediate environs. This is true for Chinese medicine as well, as long as we remember that our Medicine Wheel today is the entire planet and that we must live in the here and now. Telephones, over-night mail, and fax machines allow us access to medicine and information as quickly as riding out to the nearest medicine mountain to gather herbs once did.

Some American TCM practitioners may feel uncomfortable with some of the non-Chinese treatments I suggest herein. However, all the treatments given are based on sound TCM principles and methodology. Having to some extent mastered the Chinese materia medica, I have now broadened my vision to include a more planetary pharmacopeia. Ironically, TCM clinicians in China have for at least two decades been willing to incorporate into their treatment protocols some of the non-Chinese medicinals discussed in this book.

Therefore, besides presenting effective protocols for the treatment of cervical intraepithelial neoplasia and prostate problems and besides shedding some light on chronic viral infections in general, I hope this book will also serve as one example of a combined or integrated Chinese-Western medicine. In this New Medicine for the 21st Century, TCM supplies the theory, wisdom, and humanity, while Western science supplies more powerful and specific medicinals and therapies. I feel this approach that I am suggesting, which makes TCM theory the basis of its view, is capable of creating the kind of New Medicine our patients want.

Western medicine and the science upon which it is based tends to focus on extremely small, supposedly isolatable details. In this process, it often loses sight of the forest for the trees. Chinese medicine and the philosophy and meditational experience upon which it is based understands the impossibility of isolating anything. It, therefore, emphasizes the relationship of the part to the whole, never losing sight of the big picture. Because of this, its vision is wiser and more panoramic. It literally sees more in relationship to the whole if less than Western medicine about the small parts or pieces. From this perspective, it is the TCM practitioner who is, could, or should be the architect of the over-all treatment strategy or plan. Whereas, the Western MD is more like the carpenter or plumber who has the technical skills to make that plan a reality. This relationship between TCM practitioner and MD is similar to the relationship which currently exists between MDs and RPTs. Such a hierarchical relationship is based on an Oriental belief that the philosopher-sage should be at the helm of any endeavor, while technicians comprise the crew.

Unfortunately, up till now, attempts to combine traditional Chinese and modern Western medicines have proceeded from the other direction. Using Western science as their criteria of facticity, researchers have tried to validate traditional Chinese medicinals and therapies in its light. They have searched for the "active ingredients" in Chinese herbs and have added these herbs or these ingredients to Western medicine's pharmacopeia for the treatment of Western disease categories. This has often been done in disregard of millennia of Chinese empirical experience with these medicinals prescribed on the basis of TCM diagnosis. Such reductionism has been mostly to the detriment of modern TCM and stands capable of completely eviscerating this system of which its theory is its most important part. This theory is more holistic and wiser than Western medical theory and so is superior in the sense that Chinese medical theory can encompass Western medical theory but not *vice versa*.

Probably as much as 15 percent of the medicinals found in such modern TCM pharmacopeias as Bensky & Gamble's *Chinese Herbal Medicine: Materia Medica* were originally derived from non-Chinese sources. The Chinese themselves have, over the centuries, incorporated medicinals from all over the world into their medicine. However, in each instance, they developed a Chinese theory and methodology for their use. Our modern Medicine Wheel is made up of anything we can order by phone or fax, have delivered by over-night or express mail, and pay for by Visa or Mastercard. American practitioners of TCM would do well to keep pace with the times in which we live and master the possibilities.

This book has been written and published as a professional discussion directed at licensed health care practitioners and more specifically at those of TCM. It is not a self-help manual intended for the lay reader. Laypersons with any of the disease conditions discussed in this book are recommended to seek qualified professional care. Although this book contains information about the preventive treatment of cervical and prostate problems through diet, exercise, and deep relaxation which can be useful to lay readers, herbs are medicines and should only be prescribed remedially based on an individual, professional diagnosis, albeit a TCM diagnosis.

I encourage practitioners utilizing the protocols given in this book to send me their experiences and feedback. Works such as this are always in progress. May we all progress together towards the alleviation of the diseases of our time.

TABLE OF CONTENTS

Acknowledgements v

Foreword vii

Table of Contents xiii

Chapter One
Western Medicine & Cervical Dysplasia 1

Chapter Two
CIN, HPV, & TCM 27

Chapter Three
**The Remedial TCM Treatment of Cervical
Intraepithelial Neoplasia** 51

Chapter Four
**Complications Encountered During Remedial Treatment
Of CIN** 99

Chapter Five
The Preventive Treatment of CIN During Remission ....
.... 129

Chapter Six
The TCM Diagnosis & Treatment of Genital Warts ... 171

Chapter Seven
**Prostatitis, Prostatic Hypertrophy, and Prostate
Cancer** 187

Chapter Eight
Traditional Chinese Medicine & Prostate Problems ... 201

Chapter Nine
The Preventive Treatment of Prostate Problems 211

Chapter Ten
The Remedial TCM Treatment of Prostate Problems .. 233

Conclusion 257

Appendix I: Clinical Stages in Carcinoma of the Uterine Cervix 261

Appendix II: 263

Appendix III: Naturopathic Treatment Schedule For Escharotic Therapy In CIN 269

Appendix IV: Dietary Considerations For Candidiasis . 271

Appendix V: Pygeum Africanum 275

Appendix VI: Distributors of Medicinals Described In Text 277

Endnotes 279

Index 295

CHAPTER ONE
WESTERN MEDICINE & CERVICAL DYSPLASIA

Cervical dysplasia is the presence of abnormal cells in the cervix. It is not erosion of the cervical epithelium but rather a surface cell change. Patches of friable or secretory columnar cells replace the usual, tougher squamous cell layer of the cervix. These cells have enlarged nuclei and are hyperchromatic.[1] Cervical dysplasia is regarded as a precursor to cervical cancer or carcinoma in situ (CIS). The mean time in untreated patients to go from mild dysplasia to carcinoma in situ is 86 months. The mean time in untreated patients to go from severe dysplasia to carcinoma in situ is 12 months.[2] In fact, based on the work of Ralph M. Richart, professor of pathology at Columbia University, it is not possible to objectively identify two separate diseases -- cervical dysplasia and carcinoma in situ. Rather, this is a single continuum now referred to as cervical intraepithelial neoplasia (CIN).[3] Each year, nearly half a million women worldwide develop cervical cancer. Nearly 50% of all women who have cervical cancer die within 2 1/2 years of diagnosis.[4] A number of Western MDs, such as Richard Reid, associate professor of gynecology and obstetrics at Wayne State University School of Medicine, believe that cervical cancer is becoming more aggressive in young women[5] and that the meantime in developing CIS from dysplasia is decreasing. Therefore, the detection and early treatment of cervical dysplasia is extremely important.

In Western medicine, cervical dysplasia is diagnosed through Pap smears, colposcopies, and biopsies. The Pap smear or Papanicolaou test is the initial screening test. It consists of taking a scraping of cervical cells, staining them, and examining these cells under a microscope. If an irregularity appears on a Pap smear, then a colposcopy and a tissue biopsy may be ordered for further diagnostic evaluation. A colposcopy is the examination of the cervix by well lighted, stereoscopic magnification. It is used to identify alterations in the cervical epithelium and abnormal vascularization which regularly accompanies invasive cervical cancer. A biopsy is the taking of a snippet of tissue to also observe under microscopic inspection. However, this larger tissue sample allows for more thorough cytological examination. There are two types of cervical biopsy: the endocervical curettage and the punch biopsy. The first takes a slice of tissue from the endocervical canal. The second takes a core sample of tissue from the cervix. These tests allow for a staging in the progression of cervical dysplasia into carcinoma in situ. Modern Western medicine differentiates three basic stages of cervical dysplasia. These are:

Minimal to moderate dysplasia -
This means that there are abnormal cells in the lower 1/3 of the epithelium.

Severe dysplasia -
This means that 2/3 of the epithelium shows abnormal cells. This typically progresses to carcinoma in situ if left untreated.

Carcinoma in situ -
The full thickness of the cervical epithelium contains abnormal cells.

When cancer cells penetrate the basement membrane and invade the stroma, they can spread to adjacent pelvic organs or can be disseminated throughout the body via the lymphatic system. Such invasion of the basement membrane by malignant cells is referred to as invasive cancer of the cervix.

PAP SMEAR CLASSIFICATIONS

Most women seeking help from American TCM practitioners for the treatment of cervical dysplasia or CIN, come with an already established Western medical diagnosis. Typically, this is based on their latest Pap smear. Therefore, Western practitioners need to be familiar with these tests and the classification of their findings.

Class I - No abnormal cells, a negative Pap, suggests no problems

Class II - Atypical cells, usually due to inflammation

Class III - Cells suspicious of carcinoma

Class IV - Carcinoma in situ

Class V - Invasive cancer of the cervix

There is also another classification system in use for Pap smear results which uses a different nomenclature. It refers to the entire continuum from cervical dysplasia to cervical cancer as cervical intraepithelial neoplasia (CIN). Based on this system, a Class III Pap is further subdivided into CIN 1 and CIN 2. CIN 1 stands for mild dysplasia and CIN 2 stands for moderate dysplasia. A Class IV Pap is then categorized as CIN 3 and covers both severe dysplasia and carcinoma in situ (CIS). The chart below summarizes both these systems which are simultaneously in use.

Class I
Normal smear,
No abnormal cells

Class II
Atypical cells present
below the level of cervical
neoplasia

Class III　　　　　　　　　**Mild dysplasia**　　 = CIN 1
Smear contains abnormal
cells consistent with　　　　　**Moderate dysplasia** = CIN 2
dysplasia

Class IV　　　　　　　　　**Severe dysplasia**
Smear contains abnormal　　　　　　　　　　　　　= CIN 3
cells consistent with　　　　　**Carcinoma in situ**
carcinoma in situ

Class V
Smear contains abnormal
cells consistent with invasive
carcinoma of squamous cell
origin

(See Appendix I for the clinical staging of carcinoma of the uterine cervix.)

THE WESTERN MEDICAL TREATMENT OF CERVICAL DYSPLASIA, CIS, & INVASIVE CANCER OF THE CERVIX

The treatment of CIN in Western medicine is based on the physical destruction of the dysplastic or neoplastic cells. This is accomplished through cryosurgery, electrocoagulation, CO_2

laser, conization, or hysterectomy.[6] Patients with mild dysplasia are often simply retested in 3 months since mild dysplasia often spontaneously remits. However, I have had patients with mild dysplasia who had been recommended cryosurgery. Cryosurgery is the freezing of the superficial cervical epithelium causing the body to slough off these dead, dysplastic cells. In my experience, cervical dysplasia treated by cryosurgery often recurs.

Moderate dysplasia is more apt to be treated by either cryosurgery or, more recently now, laser cauterization. Recurrence rates with laser surgery range from 7.5-33%.[7] Conization or a cone biopsy is often the recommended treatment for severe dysplasia. This is the cutting of a cone-shaped core of tissue out of the cervix and up through the endocervical canal. This is done with a cold knife. For instance, Dr. Hugh R.K. Barber, author of *Manual of Gynecologic Oncology*, recommends conization, multiple biopsies, endocervical curettage, and either hot or cold cauterization for the treatment of moderate or marked dysplasia.[8] He does not suggest nor even make mention of any systemic treatment for dysplasias of any type.

Carcinoma in situ (CIS) is also treated by the same methods mentioned above including hysterectomy. Women who still hope to bear children are most often treated by conization. However, localized cancer of the cervix is usually treated by hysterectomy, either total if it is still very early or microinvasive or radical if it is more deeply invasive. Total hysterectomy involves removal of the uterus including the cervix. Radical hysterectomy involves removal of the cervix, surrounding tissues, the body of the uterus, and the adjacent lymph nodes. Some surgeons also remove the ovaries and fallopian tubes to prevent later ovarian cancer, especially if the patient is approaching or has gone through menopause. The Western medical literature also suggests hysterectomy even for a woman with moderate to severe dysplasia if the doctor feels the patient will comply poorly with a more conservative regime requiring repeated retesting.[9]

Depending upon the staging of invasive cancer of the cervix, radical hysterectomy, bilateral pelvic lymphadenectomy, radiation, and/or chemotherapy may be used. Radiotherapy for cancer of the cervix was first introduced by Margaret Cleves in 1903 and has been used ever since by Western MDs. The complications of radiation therapy of the cervix include irritations of the rectum, small intestine, and bladder; skin reactions; and hematopoietic depression. Fever may also occur. The above irritations may manifest as diarrhea, abdominal cramping, dysuria, polyuria, surface erythema, and ulcerations of the skin. Numerous chemotherapeutic agents have been tried for the treatment of invasive cervical cancer. These include cyclophosphamide (Cytoxan), melphalan (Alkeran), 5-fluorouracil (5FU), vincristine (Oncovin), methotrexate, hydroxyurea (Hydrea), porfiromycin, adriamycin, and bleomycin (Blenoxane). However, the results of chemotherapy as a treatment for invasive cancer of the cervix have not been favorable due to these medicinals' toxicity and exorbitant cost.[10] Only about 25-30% of cervical tumors show objective regression using these chemotherapeutics.[11]

The Western allopathic treatment of CIN is concentrated on destroying the dysplastic cells. These are either frozen, burned, or cut away. As mentioned above, cervical dysplasia treated by cryosurgery often recurs. I have seen a number of patients who had had two or more cryosurgeries and who had dysplasia once again. In addition, cryosurgery can cause cervical scarring thus rendering fertilization difficult. This is a concern among patients of childbearing age who still hope to have children. Hysterectomy obviously puts an end to all possibilities of having children. In addition, according to Chinese medical theory, hysterectomy can cause an increased probability of tumor formation due to Stagnant Blood in other, related areas of the body.

Laser surgery does offer great promise in the medicine of the future due to its low causation of trauma and scarring to the body's surrounding tissue. But, laser surgery does not nor can it redress the internal environmental factors which allow for the proliferation of dysplastic cells according to Chinese medicine. Even if laser surgery could treat cervical dysplasia in such a way that there were no recurrence, still Chinese medical treatment would be useful to correct the contributory imbalances a Western diagnosis of dysplasia suggests.

THE WESTERN ETIOLOGIES OF CERVICAL DYSPLASIA

1) Early first intercourse and/or multiple sexual partners

There is a statistical correspondence between early first intercourse and/or multiple sexual partners with increased incidence of cervical dysplasia. It is assumed that early first intercourse is associated with more sexual partners and this in turn suggests that cervical dysplasia is in some way or part a venereal or sexually transmitted disease (STD). This opinion is confirmed by Muñoz *et al.*: "The independent effect of the number of partners, and the increased risk for women whose husbands reported multiple sexual partners strongly suggests the role of a sexually transmitted infectious agent..."[12] Further, it has been shown that there is a threefold increase in incidence of cervical carcinoma among wives whose husbands had been previously married to women with cervical cancer when compared to controls.[13] Dr. Barber states that, "Among nuns and virgins cervical cancer is rare."[14] In addition, it has been noted epidemiologically that female members of religious sects which practice strict female chastity, such as Muslims and

Orthodox Jews, also have a very low incidence of cervical cancer.[15]

2) Viral infection

There are also statistical correspondences between herpes genitalia (HSV II) and human papilloma virus (HPV) infection and increased incidence of cervical dysplasia. Since these are venereal diseases, this fact supports the thesis that CIN is in some way an STD. Although there is some debate in the Western scientific literature about the causal relationship between herpes genitalia and cervical dysplasia and relatively more emphasis is currently placed on HPV, the majority of my cervical dysplasia patients do have a history of herpes genitalia even if it is seemingly latent at the time of their dysplasia. Although whole HSV II viruses have not yet been found within tumor cells, HSV II DNA, messenger RNA, and viral proteins have been found in cervical carcinoma cells. Further, Nelson et al. state that:

> An HSV-2 antigen, AG-4, has been identified by Aurelian and associates in 90 percent of cervical carcinoma biopsies, compared to 10 percent of matched control biopsies. Ninety-one percent of patients with invasive cervical carcinoma have been shown to carry antibodies to the specific antigen, compared to nine percent in matched controls. In carcinoma in situ, antibodies are detected in 68 percent of patients versus five percent in matched controls.[16]

Again according to Muñoz et al.:

> For over twenty years, much attention was focused on herpes simplex type 2, but its role in cervical neoplasia has never been adequately

confirmed or refuted. The currently favored hypothesis is that certain types of human papillomavirus (HPV) play a key aetiological role.[17]

What the Western literature is suggesting more an more is that cervical dysplasia is almost, if not always associated with human papilloma virus infection. HPV is the human wart virus. The hypothesis that HPV is a key etiological factor in cervical dysplasia, first advanced by Hansen *et al.* in 1974, has been supported by experimental data. However, it has been difficult for Western researchers to test this hypothesis epidemiologically due to difficulty in assessing HPV exposure. So far, it has not been possible to grow HPV *in vitro* nor to develop a reliable serological test for its antigens. To date, there have been more than 60 varieties of HPV identified through DNA typing. Of these, types 6 and 11 are associated with benign, condylomatous lesions and low grade dysplasia. Whereas, types 16 and 18 have been linked to cervical cancer. In all, approximately 1/3 of HPV strains have been found in anogenital tract lesions. Some doubt has recently been cast on the role of HPV in cervical cancer by reports of a high incidence of HPV 16 and 18 in normal cervical tissue. However, as Ferenczy *et al.* state, "Papillomavirus is frequently present in clinically and histologically normal cutaneous epithelium adjacent to condylomatous or intraepithelial neoplasia..."[18] This fact suggests, as Larsen *et al.* also believe, "that a latent infection stage also exists."[19] Therefore, the fact that many women may be infected with HPV 16 and 18 without current cases of cervical cancer does not rule out the possibility that they will develop dysplasia in the future.

The evidence which supports a strong etiological link between HPV and cervical cancer has been summarized by Larsen *et al.* as follows:

1) In 80% of all cervical (and penile) carcinomas, it is possible

to detect DNA of certain HPV types, usually 16 and 18, but also 31, 33, 35, 52, or 56.

2) The same virus types are found in cancers of other tissues, specifically of the anogenital region, the nasopharyngeal cavity, the tongue, and esophagus. These sites suggest a venereal transmission of these viruses through oral, anal, and genital sex.

3) These same viruses can also be found in transformed cell lines derived from these carcinomas.

4) Other types of HPV have been closely implicated with skin cancer, epidermodysplasia verruciformis (EV), and Bowen's disease.

5) Virus specific RNA has been detected *in vitro* and *in vivo*.

6) The viral proteins E6 and E7 have been identified in cell lines and in cell stages of cervical lesion development.

7) It has long been known that animal papilloma viruses are both transforming *in vitro* and tumorigenic *in vivo*.[20]

Over the years, many sexually transmitted agents have been suspected of being etiological factors in cervical dysplasia and cervical cancer. These include spermatozoa, smegma, Chlamydia Trachomatis, Neisseria Gonorrhoeae, Trichomonas Vaginalis, and Treponema Pallidum besides Herpes Simplex II. Except for the first two, all the rest are known venereal pathogens and it may be that a number of these occurring simultaneously are what cause dysplasia. If so, my guess is that it is some combination of HPV, HSV II, and/or vaginal candidiasis. Zur Hausen and Fenoglio have suggested a synergistic relationship between HPV and HSV II which may enhance the development of at least some genital tract tumors.[21] Likewise, Lancaster and Jenson state:

> The continuous exposure of these persistent lesions (i.e. HPV infections) to other factors, such as carcinogens found in tobacco products or perhaps a genital herpes virus infection or coinfection with another HPV (strain) could stimulate the proliferation of basal cells within a benign lesion. These cellular changes could arise from alterations of cellular genes, such as the activation of oncogenes or the mutation or trans-activation of the HPV genome, resulting in a progression to neoplasia.[22]

John W. Sixbey et al., in an article entitled "A Second Site for Epstein Barr Virus Shedding: The Uterine Cervix" published in *The Lancet* in 1986, suggest that Epstein-Barr virus or EBV may also be an etiological factor in CIN. "The discovery of EBV shedding in its cell-free infectious form from the uterine cervix raises the possibility of venereal transmission, neonatal infection, and EBV involvement in cervical pathology."[23] I.S. Bevan et al., in a letter to the editor also appearing in *The Lancet*, state that they found HPV DNA in the cervices of all 36 women studied with CIN. HSV DNA was found in 11, EBV DNA in 12, and HPV with either HSV or EBV DNA was found in 19. 4 of these 36 women with CIN had all three types of viral DNA.[24] As Bevan et al. state, "The finding of more than one sexually transmitted oncogenic virus in cytological material from women with histologically confirmed epithelial abnormalities suggests the need for caution when imputing aetiological significance to any one of them." R.T. Javier et al., writing in *Science*, describe their research which indicates the potentiating effects of two different strains of viruses resulting in more serious disease than either strain typically causes alone. "These results show that 2 avirulent HSV-1 variants may interact in vivo to produce virulent recombinants and a lethal infection."[25] All this suggests that more than one virus may be involved in the etiology of CIN and that two or more viruses may potentize each other causing more serious disease.

However, HPV is such an important etiological factor that we will discuss its natural history and epidemiology further below.

3) Smoking

Smokers have a 2-3 times increased incidence of cervical dysplasia.

4) Oral contraceptives

There is a well documented statistical increase in cervical cancer amongst those women who use or have used oral contraceptives (OCs).

THE WESTERN NUTRITIONAL FACTORS IN CIN

Research exists which suggests that certain micronutrient deficiencies also exist in most women with CIN. My assumption is that these vitamin/mineral deficiencies are associated with a decrease in the immune system's ability to maintain viral infection and expression in its latent stage. Therefore, such nutritional factors are not primary etiologies but complicating factors or co-factors allowing for viral expression. Nevertheless, attention to such complicating nutritional factors is important in the comprehensive treatment of CIN in that the rectification of these nutritional deficiencies enhances the organism's immune response.

Western naturopathic literature highlights the role of the following micronutrient deficiencies in the occurrence of CIN:[26]

1) Vitamin A & Beta-carotene deficiencies

Low serum beta-carotene levels are associated with a 3 times greater incidence of severe dysplasia.[27]

2) Vitamin C

There is a significant decrease in plasma levels of Vitamin C in patients with cervical dysplasia.[28]

3) Folic Acid

A Folic Acid deficiency is very commonly associated with oral contraceptive use.[29]

4) Pyridoxine (B_6)

One third of cervical cancer patients show decreases in B_6 levels.[30]

5) Selenium

Serum Selenium levels are inversely proportional to the incidence of *all* epithelial cancers and are also significantly lower in cervical dysplasia patients.[31,32]

6) Elevated Copper : Zinc ratio

An elevated Copper to Zinc ratio above 1.95 is a non-specific reaction to inflammation or malignancy and is of special importance in gynecological cancers.[33]

HPV, ITS WESTERN DESCRIPTION & DIAGNOSIS

CLASSIFICATION

Papilloma viruses are included in one of the two genuses of the family Papovaviridae. They are non-enveloped icosahedral capsid (72 capsomers) 45-55 nm in diameter. The genome is a double-stranded, circular DNA molecule of about 7,800-7,900 base pairs. The viral genomes of all the papilloma viruses are divided into an early and late region, with the late region coding for viral structural proteins. Genes of the early region encode proteins required for viral replication. Basically, papilloma viruses are the same shape as herpes viruses.

HPV INFECTION

Papilloma viruses induce hyperplasia of cells in the lower epithelial layers. However, formation of complete viral particles seems to be restricted to the upper layers of the epidermis. This suggests that only cells at a certain level of differentiation can support viral replication and late gene expression. Acanthosis or the development of spiny protrusions are a sign of retardation of the orderly maturation of squamous cells from the infected basal layer to outer layers of the epithelium. Koilocytotic changes may be the degenerative results of productive virus infection. When basal cells show proliferation and replace cells of the spinous layer, the lesion contains fewer mature cells and is classified CIN 1, 2, or 3 depending upon the extent of proliferative changes.

Papilloma viruses detected in the genital tract are considered to be readily transmitted by genital to genital contact. It is thought that moisture and abrasion of the epithelium enhance transmission. The identification of genital warts in the

Western medical literature dates back to at least the Greeks and Romans. The fact that these warts are induced by venereal transmission was established in 1954 when Barret *et al.* reported on 24 women with genital warts who first noticed their appearance 4-6 weeks after their husbands returned from the Far East. All the husbands admitted to sexual contact while overseas and all had recently had penile warts.[34]

It is generally believed that it takes approximately 3 weeks from initial infection before any obvious venereal warts may be discerned. However, it may take as long as 8 months or longer before the appearance of condylomata. It is also believed that small macules or papules, called sessile papules, due to HPV infection are more likely to transmit infection than long-standing, gross condylomata.[35]

RISK FACTORS IN GENITAL HPV INFECTION

The risk factors for genital HPV infection are similar to other sexually transmitted diseases (STD). These include multiple and casual sexual partners. However, in addition to these obvious factors, researchers have found that OC use within the previous 6 months, pregnancy, and immune system incompetence or suppression also put a woman at higher risk for developing genital condylomata. It has also been hypothesized that the presence of other STD may increase the risk of acquiring genital HPV. These include HSV II, Trichomonas Vaginalis, Candida Albicans, Treponema Pallidum (syphilis), and Haemophilus Ducreyi. All these pathogens inflame or ulcerate the squamous epithelium. STD which infect the columnar epithelium, possibly promoting squamous metaplasia, may also increase the risk of acquiring genital HPV. These include HSV II again, Chlamydia Trachomatis, and Neisseria Gonorrhoeae (gonorrhea).

GENETIC PREDISPOSITION & THE IMMUNE SYSTEM

It is suspected that some persons may be genetically predisposed to increased risk of HPV infection. This is evidenced by the fact that cervical cancer is found significantly more often in mothers and sisters of patients with cervical cancer than in the female members of consorts.[36] It is surmised that this clustering may reflect a genetic defect in the immune system resulting in an inability to either recognize or respond properly to HPV antigens. Further, it is known that persons suffering from epidermodysplasia verruciformis (EV) do have an inherited defect in cellular immunity. Moreover, persons treated with immunosuppressant therapy are at increased risk for genital tract neoplasia the longer their immunosuppressant therapy continues. And finally, anal and genital warts in men and cervical dysplasia in women are more common amongst persons infected with HIV (human immune deficiency virus).

LATENCY & THE IMMUNE SYSTEM

Lancaster and Jenson state that: "Ample evidence suggests that HPV infection can be latent."[37] This helps explain why cervical dysplasia often recurs when treatment is only directed at the destruction of the specifically dysplastic tissue. Most often, when cervical dysplasia recurs, it does so in tissue adjacent to the surgically treated area which previously had been cytologically normal. This coupled with the fact that the progression or activation of HPV depends upon both cellular and humoral (i.e. hormonal) immune mechanisms are significant facts in developing the TCM description of HPV advanced in the following chapter.

> It is possible that during latent infection, the immune system or some factor controlled by

> the immune system is able to maintain HPV gene expression in a state in which cellular morphology is unchanged. Once the immune system is disturbed, such as during pregnancy, the host loses control over viral gene expression, which results in activation of the viral genome and induction of cellular atypia and/or acanthosis. This hypothesis suggests the existence of a humoral factor produced by the immune system which can repress viral gene expression.[38]

Carson *et al.*, who studied phenotypes of peripheral blood T cells amongst 20 women with synchronously or metachronously occuring genital HPV infections and a control group of 20 women with normal cervices and no history of HPV, found that the former had a lower percentage of T4+ (helper) cells and a higher percentage of T8+ (suppressor) cells as compared to the control group.[39] This lower T4/T8 cell ratio is also seen in immune deficient HIV positives. Lancaster and Jenson feel that rejection of an established HPV-induced lesion is probably mediated by either a local cellular or systemic cellular response and that circulating antibodies appear to play a role in protecting against reinfection.[40] It is also felt by some researchers that HPV viral expression may be cyclic. That means that there may be some biorhythmic cyclicity to their activity as yet unspecified.

TREATMENT, RECURRENCE, & THE IMMUNE SYSTEM

As stated above, about 1/3 of cervical dysplasias treated surgically recur. Larry I. Lipshultz of the department of urology at Baylor College of Medicine states:

Cure rates for condyloma, especially subclinical condyloma, are notoriously low. Treatment efficacy for standard therapies range from 20% to 90% in the intermediate treatment period. After 3 months, however, many patients have recurrent condyloma in the same area.[41]

Evidence suggests that once a productive human papilloma virus infection has been established, trauma or surgical intervention, when it works, may enhance the regression of condylomata by stimulating the immune system, thereby leading to a more widespread distribution of viral antigens. This thus boosts the cellular and humoral immune response. If this is true, it would also suggest that the 1/3 of all patients whose condylomata recur do so because of some incompetence in their immune response. Dr. Lipshultz confirms this opinion when he says, "Because some (genital) condyloma spontaneously disappear, as do some common body warts, it is clear that a large role in the infection is played by the individual patient's cell-mediated immunity."[42]

EPIDEMIOLOGY

The number of first time visits to MDs for the treatment of genital warts in the United States has increased seven-fold from 1966 to 1984. The number of people with visible external genital warts is merely the tip of the iceberg however. There are approximately 1,000,000 cases of condylomata reported annually in the United States at present.[43] It is assumed that an additional 2,440,000 persons have subclinical genital HPV infections requiring magnification to detect. Another 20,740,000 are infected subclinically which would require DNA probes or hybridization to detect. And as many as 97,600,000 Americans between the ages of 15-49 were at risk for acquiring genital HPV infection in 1987.[44] A more conservative estimate of genital HPV infection is given by Ralph M. Richart, professor of pathology at Columbia University. In April 1989, Dr. Ferenczy estimated that "15 million North Americans either have genital HPV infections or carry HPV DNA."[45] Give or take 5 million, this is a lot of Americans infected with potentially carcinogenic viruses.

DIAGNOSIS

There are three ways a genital HPV infection can manifest and, consequently, three different categories of Western diagnostic procedures. The three categories of HPV diagnosis are 1) unaided visible detection, 2) microscopic visible detection, and 3) detection by DNA probe and/or hybridization. HPV infection resulting in gross condylomata can be identified by unaided visual inspection. There are characteristic, gross, warty lesions on the cervix, vagina, vulva, and/or anus in women and on the penis and/or anus in men. These lesions can be relatively small, cauliflower-shaped lesions similar to common body warts or can be large, irregular masses of warty, acanthotic tissue totally surrounding the vaginal and anal orifices. Such gross, visible lesions are considered the clinical manifestation of HPV infection.

The second way HPV infection may manifest is termed subclinical. This consists of small macules and sessile papules which can hardly been seen with the naked eye or which require magnification to see. Gynecologists use colposcopes to detect these subclinical lesions in women and urologists use colposcopes to detect them in men. As mentioned above, a colposcope is a microscope for examining the body stereoscopically under illumination and at various magnifications. First the area is bathed in vinegar (4.5% acetic acid). This is allowed to dry for 3-5 minutes. Then the area is examined. Areas of subclinical HPV hyperplasia will tend to stain white. This is called an aceto-white reaction. However, areas of fungal infection and areas exposed to constant friction may stain aceto-white and, therefore, give false positives. Both men and women's genitalia can thus be inspected including the inside of the vagina and the cervix itself.

The third way HPV infection may manifest is also subclinical. However, in this case, there are no visible lesions even with magnification, illumination, and aceto-white staining. This form of HPV infection can only be detected cytologically through Pap smears and HPV DNA probes and hybridization. Pap smears identify dysplastic or neoplastic cells usually before any obvious, overt pathology is present. However, HPV DNA/RNA identification techniques, such as the Southern blot test, the ViraPap, and DNA hybridization, can identify both the presence of invisible HPV and the strain of virus, whether 6, 11, 16, 18, etc. HPV DNA screening tests can be performed on both men and women. In men, a swab is taken from the urethra and a urine sample is also checked. HPV has been found in both the urine and the ejaculate. This latter technology is still very new. However, it does allow for early detection of HPV infection and also identification of those infected with the most carcinogenic strains of virus.

Some Western MDs in the forefront of research on HPV recommend that such ViraPap tests be done on a regular basis and that they should be considered a routine screening procedure in addition to the more common Pap smear. False negative Paps do occur and such ViraPaps would provide a back-up test. Thomas M. Becker, MD, assistant professor of medicine at the University of New Mexico, believes that all sexually active women should be screened for HPV if they have multiple partners.[46] Although the FDA has approved the ViraPap test, often HPV screening is only done at research and teaching hospitals and clinics. Some MDs also suggest the use of routine colposcopies for screening purposes. However, this procedure requires special equipment and training and is not cost-effective as a routine screening test. In any case, colposcopy cannot detect HPV infection which is not visible under microscopic inspection.

Suggested indications for HPV DNA testing are as follows:

1) Current or previous STD

2) Equivocal Pap smear (at any age)

3) Equivocal Pap smear despite therapy with intravaginal conjugated estrogen (after menopause)

4) History of multiple sexual partners

5) Immunocompromise

6) *In utero* exposure to DES (test during or after menopause)

7) Re-evaluation after cancer treatment

Dr. Alex Ferenczy recommends testing all men whose female partners have documented HPV infections but whose penis and/or anus contain no clinically or androscopically visible lesions.[47] Dr. Duane E. Townsend recommends that individuals testing positive for HPV 18 be followed at 4-6 month intervals instead of the usual 12 month intervals generally suggested for non-dysplastic patients.[48] Dr. Ferenczy suggests that patients testing positive for HPV 16 or 18 receive repeat Pap smear every 6 months and that those testing positive for HPV 6, 11, and 42 only be retested once per year.[49] Although there is some difference in these two doctors' timing for follow-up care, they both agree that persons testing positive for HPV 16 and 18 need to be followed and tested more frequently. This is based on the suggestion "that HPV 18 may be increasing in prevalence and may be responsible for the anecdotal increase in more rapidly progressive poorly differentiated squamous carcinomas or adenocarcinomas in young women."[50]

THE WESTERN TREATMENT OF HPV INFECTION IN WOMEN

Western medicine specifically addresses three areas of the female anatomy where HPV infection may occur. These are the cervix, the vagina, and the vulva. Since early CIN lesions are difficult to differentiate from HPV colposcopically, cyctologically, and histologically, and since most patients with CIN have areas of HPV, it is currently recommended that colposcopically visible subclinical HPV infection be treated in the same manner as CIN.[51] That means surgically, whether by cryosurgery, laser surgery, or cold knife. At the moment there is no Western allopathic therapy for subclinical, invisible HPV infection of the cervix. Women with such latent HPV infection are merely followed at more frequent than usual intervals between repeat Pap smears and colposcopy, and even this is a recent development.

Condylomatous growth pattern is commonly seen in the vagina, usually in association with vulvar condylomata. When these can be diagnosed colposcopically, there are several Western treatments for them. The first is a 50-80% solution of Bichloracetic Acid (BCA) or Trichloracetic Acid (TCA) applied topically. This treatment is limited to a few lesions at a time and is repeated weekly. The second treatment option is laser surgery. This is only useful when there are only a few localized lesions. This method is not suitable for diffuse viral disease. For diffuse condylomatous lesions, the chemotherapeutic agent 5-flourouracil (5-FU) may be used as a 5% cream applied topically. 2 grams of this are inserted high into the vagina with an intravaginal applicator once per week. This treatment can continue for a protracted period and is considered "an ideal therapy for (the) immunosuppressed host."[52] Re-examination should be scheduled at 2 week intervals.

The last standard Western treatment for vaginal HPV is Interferon injection. This is a so-called immune-modulating therapy designed to stimulate the host's own local immune response. 1,000,000 IU are injected intraoitally 3 times per week for 1 month. For those who respond, this therapy is continued once a week for an additional 8 weeks. If there is no response, a local destructive method (BCA or laser cauterization) must be used. Typically, flu-like symptoms occur as a side-effect of Interferon therapy 2-3 hours after injection which last 2-6 hours. Western MDs use Acetominophen to treat these side effects. However, according to the theory advanced below, such side-effects are evidence of the Righteous Qi's struggle with the exteriorized pathogen, and care must be taken that any treatment aimed at these symptoms not suppress this exteriorization. This exteriorization is a sign of regressive vicariation. Suppression of such symptoms of exteriorization may result in progressive or pathological vicariation.[53]

Condyloma acuminatum is the most common growth pattern on the vulva. There may be epithelial spicules or acanthosis, papilliform or cauliflower-like growth, and ulceration. The standard Western medical treatment of vulvar HPV resulting in condylomata acuminatum is first chemo-destructive using either BCA or TCA applied topically. This treatment is applied weekly as long as the lesions are regressing until they are no longer visible with the colposcope.

Unfortunately, since latent HPV is almost always present in the seemingly normal tissue adjacent to the more obvious lesions, often new warty lesions appear in those areas. After 4-6 weekly applications of BCA, those patients who present a new crop of condylomata each week are considered due to a failure of immune response. These patients are then suggested to be switched to Interferon. However, according to Dr. Lipshultz, both vaginal and vulvar condylomata tend to recur once Interferon therapy is suspended.[54]

For subclinical HPV vulvar and vaginal infections, Kenneth D. Hatch, author of *Handbook of Colposcopy: Diagnosis and Treatment of Lower Genital Tract Neoplasia and HPV Infection,* recommends Interferon injection therapy. 1,000,000 IU are injected subcutaneously into the intraoital skin near the hymenal ring 3 times per week for 1 month. After colposcopy reveals no further microscopic lesions, treatment is given once per week for another 6 weeks. If, however, symptoms persist, the Western gynecologist is suggested to consider minor vestibular gland excision.[55]

VULVAR INTREPITHELIAL NEOPLASIA (VIN)

Vulvar intraepithelial neoplasia (VIN) is related to CIN or cervical intraepithelial neoplasia in that current research suggests that both are due to HPV infection. According to Dr. Hatch:

> The incidence of VIN is increasing, and the age of the patient is decreasing. This is a result of the increased incidence of HPV infection as the majority of these lesions are HPV DNA positive.[56]

VIN tend to be whitish with a thick, hyperkeratotic layer on the epithelial surface. They may also be red with absence of hyperkeratotic layer but have nuclei retained on the surface. Or, they may be pigmented, with pigmentation from the basal layer carried to the surface by rapid epithelial proliferation. A single patient may exhibit one or all of these manifestations. Approximately 35% of VIN patients have associated intraepithelial lesions of the anogenital tract with the cervix being the most common secondary site.

Diagnosis of VIN is made using colposcopy and biopsy. Prior to 1970, VIN was treated by total vulvectomy. However, now this is considered gross over-treatment. There are two current standard Western treatments for VIN. The first is local surgical excision. This is recommended when there are focal lesions on redundant vulvar skin which can be easily re-approximated or when further diagnostic studies are needed, i.e. biopsied tissue. Laser vaporization is performed on multiple lesions or lesions covering a large area. It is also used when lesions involve the clitoris or anus. Again unfortunately, recurrence is common, occuring in approximately 20% of patients. Therefore, Western MDs recommend colposcopic re-examination of the entire anogenital tract every 6 months.

Genital warts were once considered a bothersome but negligible problem with no long-term negative health consequences. This is no longer the common wisdom on HPV. HPV infection is implicated in an increased incidence of neoplasia of the anogenital tract and HPV DNA has even been found in metastatic ovarian and liver tumors.[57] It is becoming more and more obvious that HPV infection is both widely disseminated in the young adult and middle-aged American population and poses a serious health threat.

From the TCM point of view, the allopathic or modern Western medical treatment of CIN and HPV infection are not totally satisfactory. Even the latest edition of *The Merck Manual* plainly states that for HPV infection no modern Western medical treatment is completely satisfactory.[58] Either its therapies are prone to relapse, themselves cause irreversible iatrogenesis, or do not address the underlying causes of the occurrence of dysplasia. However, Western epidemiology does tell us more about cervical dysplasia than is immediately evident by TCM alone, and Pap smears do provide an early warning that something is seriously amiss before TCM diagnosis is, in most cases, able.

On the other hand, TCM theory provides more insight into all the factors which cause CIN and, based on these insights, can provide safer, more comprehensive, but nonetheless effective therapy. Additionally, patients undergoing such comprehensive TCM treatment for CIN and HPV infection experience a rebalancing in their total metabolism which benefits their health in many other areas besides their cervices.

By combining the best of modern Western medicine and Traditional Chinese Medicine, we can supply a superior treatment for cervical intraepithelial neoplasia which not only addresses the major complaint but restores better health to the entire organism. However, before we can do that, we must first come up with a TCM description of CIN and HPV.

CHAPTER TWO
CIN, HPV, & TCM

Cervical dysplasia is not a traditional Chinese disease category. There is no one Chinese disease category which covers identically cervical dysplasia. Nor are Pap smears one of the Four (Methods of Chinese) diagnosis. Pap smear findings cannot automatically be translated into any one TCM Pattern (of Disharmony or *Zheng*). What then should a TCM practitioner do when faced with a patient whose main complaint is cervical dysplasia?

1) Do a straight TCM diagnosis by *Bian Zheng*. *Bian Zheng* means the discrimination of professionally categorized Patterns (of Disharmony). Diagnosis by *Bian Zheng* is the hallmark and definition of TCM methodology. Of the three things the TCM practitioner should do as described herein, it is the most important. Without an individualized diagnosis by *Bian Zheng*, there is no TCM.[1]

2) Look at TCM descriptions of the disease mechanisms of cervical cancer and work backward. Since cervical dysplasia becomes cervical cancer if left untreated over time, the practitioner should be able to work backward from the TCM *Bian Zheng* for cervical cancer in order to gain a better understanding of the disease mechanisms (*Bing Ji*) involved. There do currently exist in English discussions of the TCM *Bian Zheng* diagnosis of cervical cancer.[2,3]

3) Think according to TCM logic and methodology about the four Western etiological factors mentioned above. If one ponders each of these four from the point of view of TCM, much further insight and information on the TCM disease mechanisms and treatment of cervical dysplasia can be gained.

Although the first piece of advice above is the single most important and essential to the TCM treatment of dysplasia, I will discuss numbers 2 and 3 first since diagnosis by *Bian Zheng* is basic to TCM education and this book is not a primer on the differentiation of signs and symptoms.

TCM DESCRIPTIONS OF CERVICAL CANCER

BIAN BING

There are two main methodologies of diagnosis in traditional Chinese medicine in its broadest sense. These are diagnosis by *Bian Bing* or the discrimination of named disease categories and diagnosis by *Bian Zheng* or the discrimination of professionally defined Patterns (of Disharmony). The first methodology is common to all styles of Chinese medicine. The second, diagnosis by *Bian Zheng*, is specifically the hallmark of TCM as a particular style of Chinese medicine.

Cervical cancer is not a traditional Chinese *Bing* or named category of disease. Rather, cervical cancer is a Western medical category of disease. However, Zhang Dai-Zhao, in *The Treatment of Cancer by Integrated Chinese-Western Medicine*[4], states that if one looks at the first early signs of cervical cancer as diagnosed by the Four (Methods of) diagnosis, these fall into two traditional Chinese disease categories:

1) *Dai Xia*

2) *Beng Lou*

Dai Xia means morbid or abnormal vaginal discharge. Classically, *Dai Xia* is subdivided into the *Wu Dai* or Five *Dai*: White, Yellow, Red, Green, and Black. This five-fold classification is based on Five Phase theory and correspondences. However, in modern TCM gynecology, *Dai Xia* is divided into three subcategories: *Bai Dai* (White Discharge), *Huang Dai* (Yellow Discharge), and *Chi Bai Dai* (Red & White Discharge). Although there are a number of disease mechanisms accounting for all the various types of *Dai Xia*, in clinical practice, the most common cause of *Dai Xia* is Damp Heat which can account for species of White, Yellow, and Red & White *Dai*. Persistent *Huang Dai* or Yellow Discharge is especially suggestive of cervical cancer and *Huang Dai* is always due to Dampness and Heat.

Beng Lou means abnormal vaginal bleeding. In Chinese, it is a compound term. *Beng* means avalanche or flooding. *Lou* means a persistent leak or trickle. *Beng Lou* can either refer to menorrhagia which continues beyond the normal span of the period or is excessively heavy or to metrorrhagia which is bleeding at other than during the period. Although there are a number of TCM disease mechanisms accounting for all the various species of *Beng Lou*, in clinical practice here in the United States, the most common disease mechanism is Heat causing the Blood to run recklessly outside its *Dao* or Pathways.

Jia Kun, in *The Prevention and Treatment of Carcinoma in Traditional Chinese Medicine*, expands upon the earliest signs and symptoms of cervical cancer.[5] He lists:

1) Irregular vaginal bleeding

2) Spotting after coitus

3) Increased *Dai Xia*

4) Lower abdominal pain

5) A red or dark purple tongue, swollen tongue, red spots or *Dian*, and a white or yellow coating

6) A slippery fast, thready fast, deep fast, or thready wiry pulse

The first two of these symptoms correspond to the Chinese disease category *Beng Lou*. However, in my experience, women with cervical dysplasia often have early periods. This is the disease category or Chinese *Bing* called *Yue Jing Xian Qi*, Moon Flow Before Schedule. In the majority of clinically encountered cases, *Yue Jing Xian Qi* is due to some species of Evil Heat, most frequently Depressive Liver Heat.

Increased *Dai Xia* we have already discussed. Lower abdominal pain is the disease category *Shao Fu Tong* in Chinese medicine. In women, *Shao Fu Tong* most often occurs in relationship to the period, in which case it is referred to as *Tong Jing*, Painful Flow or dysmenorrhea. In my experience, the most common disease mechanism in American women for *Shao Fu Tong* and *Tong Jing* is Stagnant Qi and Blood with Mutual Entanglement of Damp Heat.[6]

The tongue and pulse signs we will discuss under *Bian Zheng*. However, in reviewing the traditional Chinese *Bing* or disease categories accounting for the earliest stages of cervical cancer, the most commonly encountered disease mechanisms associated with these Chinese diseases are Dampness, Heat, and

Stagnation of Qi and Blood.

BING YIN

In Chinese TCM clinical manuals, after the statement of the named disease under discussion, the next heading is *Bing Yin*. *Bing Yin* literally means disease cause. It can be translated as either etiology or pathogenesis. Jia Kun, following standard TCM methodology, divides the *Bing Yin* of cervical cancer into Internal causes (*Nei Yin*), External causes (*Wai Yin*), and Neither Internal Nor External causes (*Bu Nei Bu Wai Yin*).[7]

The Internal cause (*Nei Yin*) of cervical cancer is *Qi Qing Nei Shang*. This means Internal Injury (due to the) Seven Passions. Basic TCM theory allows us to elaborate on Jia Kun's statement. First of all, emotional disturbances cause disruption in the flow and patency of the Qi. Since the Qi moves the Blood and Body Fluids, emotional upset can indirectly effect these as well. Secondly, the Seven Passions tend to transform into Heat. Any strong emotional upset may cause Internal Accumulation of Evil Heat. And third, the Organ foremost effected by emotional disturbance is the Liver. This is because it is the Liver's function to maintain the free flow and patency of the Qi. If the Qi flow becomes disturbed, this, in turn, will effect the Liver. In TCM, it is, therefore, said that the Liver is the temperamental Organ. Further, when the Qi flow in the Liver is disturbed, it becomes stuck or congested. It is also said in Chinese medicine that the Liver tends to Excess. Stuck Qi is Excess locally. Typically, this Excess or Repletion becomes Hot based on Liu Wan-su's Principle of Similar Transformation.

Jia Kun also says that the Six Evils, the *Liu Xie*, may also contribute to the causation of cervical cancer. These are the External causes or *Wai Yin*. This means that CIN can be "caught" from an outside source, that one can be invaded from the outside. Although TCM texts talk of Six Evils, since the 17th and 18th Centuries, the concept of *Li Qi*, Epidemic or Pestilential Qi, has been added to the Chinese discussion of External causes. *Li Qi* accounts for epidemic, transmissible diseases from person to person. Wu You-ke, author of the *Wen Yi Lun* (*The Theory of Plague*), said, "One disease, one Qi." This means that *Li Qi* cause specific, similar diseases in all infected persons. This is very similar to Western germ theory. Further, Chinese medical theory also says regarding *Li Qi* that it will tend to invade all persons it comes in contact with regardless of the strength of their *Wei Qi* and regardless of the *Wu Yun Liu Qi* (the Five Transports/Six Qi). This latter theory describes the cyclic relationship of the Six Evils to biorhythms and weather. As we will see below, the External causes of cervical dysplasia and, therefore, cervical cancer include *Li Qi* Evils introduced from outside.

Jia Kun mentions that both Internal Injury from the Seven Passions and External Invasion by the Six Evils can cause Stagnation of the Qi, Blood, Food, Dampness, Phlegm, and Fire. These are Zhu Dan-xi's Six Stagnations which are all mutually co-productive. However, it is the Qi which transports and transforms all of these and, therefore, Stagnation of Qi is especially important as a disease mechanism or *Bing Ji*.

As for *Bu Nei Bu Wai Yin*, Jia Kun adds Injury to the *Chong* and *Ren* due to sex shortly after delivery. Delivery and the postpartum lochia are energetically analogous to a large period during which the flow of Blood is down and out. Sexual intercourse causes a reversal in this flow upwards and in. This, in turn, causes a collision, as it were, resulting in the formation of Stagnant Blood. However, there are other things which may also cause Stagnant Blood and, therefore, Qi, Heat, and Dampness. These include sex during menstruation, sex too soon after abortions, abortions themselves, and IUDs, to name some common American *Bu Nei Bu Wai Yin*. In addition, under *Bu Nei Bu Wai Yin* are also listed *Chong*. *Chong* literally means insect or worm, but also means any "creepy crawler", such as toads, snakes, scorpions, etc. As we will see below, at least one species of *Chong*, *Zhen Jun* or yeast, also participates in the etiology of many American women's CIN.

If we summarize this discussion of *Bing Yin*, we come up with Stagnation & Accumulation, Heat, and Dampness to which we must add Pestilential or *Li Qi* and parasites or *Chong*.

TCM REFLECTIONS ON THE 4 WESTERN ETIOLOGIES OF CERVICAL DYSPLASIA

We have seen above that Western medicine posits four possible etiological factors causing or participating in the cause of cervical dysplasia. The first is early and/or multiple sexual partners. This, as we have mentioned, suggests that cervical dysplasia is an STD. In TCM, this suggests that, as Jia Kun states, cervical dysplasia is in part due to some External pathogens. Since these pathogens are transmitted from person to person, I think we can further say that they are a species of *Li Qi*, and, when we talk about *Li Qi* in Chinese medicine, that immediately implies that the disease is a species of *Wen Bing*. We will return to this line of reasoning momentarily.

Secondly, we have seen that both the herpes simplex virus II (HSV II) and the human papilloma virus (HPV) are strongly implicated in cervical dysplasia. Both of these are known to be transmitted through sexual contact and are species of venereal disease. This bolsters both the fact that External pathogens play a part in cervical dysplasia and that these pathogens are a *Li Qi* of the *Wen Bing* category.

Third, smoking is statistically related to a higher than average incidence of cervical dysplasia. In the late 19th Century, Jin

Zi-jou wrote a description of the negative impact of smoking on the organism according to Chinese medical theory.

> Tobacco has a Dry, Bitter energy which most easily damages the Qi and attacks the Lungs. When the Lungs are injured, Qi loses its clearing and dispersing (ability) and the Yellow Bell loses its resonance.[8]

The Lungs control the Liver. If the Lungs lose their ability to disperse and clear the Qi, then the Liver is allowed to become Excess and impatent. It is the Liver Meridian which primarily irrigates and circulates the genitalia and Uterus. If the Lungs do not control the Liver by adequately dispersing its Qi, symptoms of Stagnation and Heat can arise anywhere along the Liver Channel's course. In women, such signs often manifest in the genitalia and Uterus.

In addition, smoking tobacco causes persistent Heat to accumulate in the Lungs. This causes a tendency for the Heart, which participates with the Lungs in the *Zong* or Chest Qi, to also become Hot. This Heat is transferred to the Heart Blood and thence to the Liver which stores the Blood. At the same time, the Dry, Hot nature of smoking tobacco causes an exhaustion of Lung Yin which, in turn, over time exhausts the Kidney Yin as well.

Most smokers use smoking to unconsciously disperse and scatter stuck Qi since tobacco itself is dispersing. However, the long-term effects of this unskillful method of dealing with Qi Congestion are, in the end, counterproductive and deleterious.

And fourth, oral contraceptive use is also statistically related to an increased incidence of cervical dysplasia. I have described at some length elsewhere the TCM effects of OCs on the human organism. However, in sum, their effects are to cause Stagnation of Qi and Blood at the same time as they waste the Blood and *Jing*. We have seen above that Stagnation of Qi and Blood do play a part in the TCM description of cervical dysplasia. In addition, Stagnation of Qi and Blood can cause Excess Heat, and Exhaustion of Blood and *Jing* Essence allows the activation and flourishing of Pestilential, Hidden Hot Toxins.

WEN BING XUE

Next, we must discuss *Wen Bing Xue* or Warm Disease theory before we can understand the disease mechanisms responsible for cervical dysplasia as thoroughly as possible. Warm Disease theory was developed in the 1600 and 1700s by Ye Tian-shi and Wu Ju-tong in response to the rise in epidemic, pestilential diseases in turn due to the rise of densely populated cities. In the face of cholera, typhus, typhoid, bubonic plague, and diphtheria, Zhang Zhong-qing's *Shang Han* theory was insufficient and not perfectly applicable.

Already in the Jin-Yuan Dynasties, Liu Wan-su, based on a line in the *Nei Jing*, had developed the idea that most human disease is due to pathological Heat. Liu Wan-su created out of this observation the School of Cold and Cool (Medicine, *Han Liang Pai*), many of whose remedies are still effective for the treatment of acute viral diseases such as influenza. However, Ye Tian-shi and Wu Ju-tong systematized the progression of a Warm Evil Disease similar to how Zhang Zhong-qing had systematized the progression of a Cold Injury, and thus they created a sophisticated differential diagnosis and an effective treatment protocol for dealing with such epidemic, pestilential diseases. This theory continued to be refined throughout the 18th and 19th Centuries and is still being refined to this day.

According to *Wen Bing Xue*, a Warm Evil progresses through the organism in successive stages or layers. These stages are called the *Si Fen* or Four Stages in contradistinction to Zhang Zhong-qing's Six *Fen*. The Four *Fen* are the *Wei Fen, Qi Fen, Ying Fen,* and *Xue Fen*. Typically, a Warm Evil first enters the outermost or most superficial layer, the *Wei Fen*, and then works its way inward. At each stage, there are specific, characteristic signs and symptoms allowing for differential diagnosis and treatment. Through proper treatment, a Warm Evil may be stopped or negated at any stage or the course of a disease through these four stages may be speeded up and made less severe. It is also possible for a Warm Evil to skip one or more stages or to progress contrary to the scheme outlined above.

In addition, it was also recognized that typically *Wen Bing* progress from the Upper Burner during their most superficial stage (effecting the Lungs) to the Middle Burner (effecting the Stomach) and finally to the Lower Burner (effecting the Kidney/Bladder, Large Intestine, and Uterus). However, this progression may skip Burners and may even progress in the opposite direction. *The Revised Outline of Traditional Chinese Medicine* specifically says that it is *Fu Xie*, Hidden Evils or latent pathogens, which progress from Inside to Outside and from Bottom to Top.[9]

Venereal diseases in TCM are species of *Wen Bing*. Since CIN seems to be a venereal disease, it too, in part, should be approached as a *Wen Bing*. However, there is one more peculiarity that must be discussed in terms of the Warm External Evil which contributes to the development of CIN. In Chinese medicine, there is the concept of *Fu Xie* mentioned above. This literally means Hidden Evil but is also often translated as latent pathogen. Hidden Evils are first discussed in the *Nei Jing* where it says that an invading External pathogen may remain hidden or latent within the body to be activated at some later time when the Internal environment is conducive to its flourishing.[10] The External pathogens responsible for venereal diseases, such as syphilis, herpes genitalia, chlamydia, cervical dysplasia, and AIDS, are all species of *Fu Xie* or Hidden Evils of the *Wen Re*, Warm Hot variety. In Chinese, such pathogens are called *Wen Fu Xie Qi*, Warm Hidden Evil Qi or Warm Hidden Evils for short.

All of the STD mentioned above typically enter the Lower Burner first and immediately lodge in the *Xue Fen* or Blood Phase where they remain latent or hidden. Wu Ju-tong's theory of a *Wen Xie*'s progression through the Three Burners specifically describes Damp Heat in each of these Burners. Therefore, saying that the pathogens associated with STD enter or lodge in the Lower Burner implies that these pathogens are Damp as well as Hot. Although Damp Heat does not typically invade the *Ying* and *Xue Fen*, according to Liu Yan-chi, it can.[11] This is more likely if Heat predominates over Dampness. Severe Heat tends to injure the Blood, but persistent Heat wastes the Yin. While Dampness impedes the Yang. In the Lower Burner, this means Kidney Yang and Large Intestine Qi. If the Heat is Excess enough, it can cause reckless flow of Blood outside its *Dao* or Pathways. But persistent, low-grade Heat causes depletion of Yin Humor and a *Zheng Qi* Deficiency. In the case of HIV, there may be an initial, short-lived *Wei Fen* stage, but often either this goes unrecognized or is absent. Likewise, in herpes genitalia and syphilis, there may be localized, Damp, Hot lesions immediately after invasion or infection, or, as with chlamydia and HPV, the Warm Evils may immediately go latent only to arise as active symptomology at some later date.

Drs. Wu Bo-ping and Lu Shou-kang of the Chinese Academy of TCM in Beijing point out in relationship to AIDS that it is the decline of Kidney Essence which allows for the activation of a *Fu Xie* or Hidden Evil. "The crucial point in the prevention of *Wen Bing* is the tight storage of Kidney Essence."[12] This is based on the *Nei Jing* stating: "The Essence is the Root of the body; for those who have it (well) stored (in Winter), Warm Diseases may not occur in Spring."[13]

When venereal *Fu Xie* go from hidden or latent to active, they typically can be described as Damp Heat diseases since their most distinctive signs and symptoms tend to be a combination of Dampness and Heat. It is my clinical experience that not only a lessening of Kidney *Jing* but also an increase in Dampness and Heat Internally and in particular in the Lower Burner combine to allow the flourishing of such venereal Warm Hidden Evils such as HPV and HSV II. This is corroborated by the following statement by Jia Kun regarding cervical papilloma : "Cervical papilloma occurs mostly during pregnancy with cauliflower (i.e. wart-like) shape, causing vaginal bleeding and increased leukorrhea and disappears by itself after delivery."[14]

I myself know of two such cases, one in China and one in the United States. During pregnancy, the woman's Blood and Jing are used to nourish the growing fetus. This puts a strain on and can deplete the mother's Blood and *Jing*, which it is said in TCM share a common source -- the Kidneys. Likewise, during pregnancy, there is a downward drive of Heat and Body Fluids. Blood itself is Warm and the Heart sends the Blood down to the *Bao Gong* to nourish the fetus via the *Bao Mai*. Blood and Body Fluids share a common source and both are transported by the Qi. As the Blood is focused downward, so Body Fluids also travel along, accentuating the normal tendency of Dampness to percolate downward. This, as Jia Kun points out, can cause in some women, i.e. those infected with HPV, the development of *Dai Xia* and *Tai Lou*, Fetal Leakage, and the growth of wart-like neoplasms on their cervix. After delivery, with the recuperation of their *Jing* and reversal of flow of the *Chong Mai/Bao Mai* thus dissipating the

Dampness and Heat in their Lower Burner, the wart-like neoplasm may often spontaneously disappear. This means, in TCM terms, the Warm Evil becomes hidden or latent again.

Therefore, if in fact HPV and HSV II can cause cervical dysplasia and if HPV and HSV II can be described in TCM as *Wen Fu Xie Qi*, then two important considerations for the prevention and treatment of cervical dysplasia arise:

1) Maintenance of the Kidney *Jing* at healthy levels and prevention of accumulation of Damp Heat in the Lower Burner in the hidden or latent stage, and

2) Dissolution of Damp Heat Toxins and tonification of the *Jing* Essence during the active stage.

In other words, anything which exhausts or wastes the *Jing* Essence on the one hand or gives rise to Dampness and Heat on the other would be prejudicial to the health of anyone infected with HPV or HSV II and in women is likely to give rise to CIN.

The following is a list of factors which exhaust the *Jing* Essence according to TCM theory. This list is merely indicative and is not necessarily categorically complete.

1) Long-term fatigue

2) Continuous stress

3) Excessive sex

4) Recreational drugs

5) Aging

6) Pregnancy

7) Bleeding, including too heavy or too frequent menstruation

8) Impaired digestion, including candidiasis, amoebiasis, and worms

9) Insomnia

10) Coffee

11) Smoking

12) Chronic disease

13) Inappropriate or prolonged fasting

14) High fever

15) Stagnant Blood impeding the formation of fresh or new Blood

Factors which create Damp Heat include:

1) Wrong diet

Some foods create Excessive Heat. These include spicy, Hot, Acrid foods, chicken, and shrimp, to name just a few. Some foods create excessive Dampness: pork, beef, dairy products, too much liquids with meals, too much salad and raw fruits, and sugars and sweets. And some foods create both Dampness and Heat simultaneously: oily, greasy, fatty foods and alcohol, for instance.

2) Liver Qi

Gan Qi or Liver Qi in TCM means a pathological state of Liver Qi Congestion. Usually this is due to emotional upset and stress, although it can be aggravated by over-eating and Stagnant Food. If Liver Qi persists, it often transforms into Depressive Liver Heat or Depressive Liver Fire. This *Hua Re* or Transformative Heat may manifest anywhere along the course of the *Jue Yin*, either externally or internally. If there is Dampness percolating downward, it often becomes entangled and mutually promoting with Liver Heat which is then confined to the Lower Burner.

3) Stagnant Blood

Stagnant Blood also often transforms into Hot Stagnant Blood for the same reason that Stagnant Qi transforms into Depressive Liver Heat. Both these transformations are based on Liu Wan-su's Principle of Similar Transformation, one of the most important principles in Chinese medicine for understanding disease mechanism and evolution. This Heat can also become entangled with Dampness percolating down into the Lower Burner.

4) Lack of Exercise

Lack of exercise can cause both Dampness and Heat. Exercise circulates the Qi and Blood and dissipates Accumulation. Exercise helps redress both Stagnant Qi and Blood, thus preventing or dissipating Transformative Heat. Likewise, because exercise circulates the Qi and Qi moves Dampness and Food, adequate exercise is also important for preventing and redressing Stagnant Food and Stagnant Dampness.

5) Oral Contraceptives

Because oral contraceptives tend to engender Stagnant Qi and Stagnant Blood, they also can cause or aggravate any accumulation of Transformative Heat. Although they tend to wither the Blood, Transformative Heat arising from Stagnant Qi and Stagnant Blood may become entangled with Dampness percolating down from the Middle Burner.

In Chinese medicine, it is believed that Heat and Dampness are mutually co-productive. Heat can stew the Juices which, when they condense, can become Dampness. And Dampness, being Yin, can impede the flow of Qi which is Yang, thus causing Transformative Heat. A certain amount of Dampness and Heat are usually produced as one ages. These tend to accumulate to the point where they cause pathologies in the 40s and 50s and into the 60s and 70s. As a person ages, Excess Heat typically transforms into Deficiency Heat. In such cases, the Heat is Deficiency Heat and the Dampness is Excess. Such mixed Excess/Deficiency Damp Heat is characterized by its low but persistent level of inflammation.

Latent Vs. Hidden

Fu Xie literally means Hidden Evil. The *Fu* in this case is the same as in *Fu Mai*, a hidden pulse, and *Fu Ling*, Hidden Paper-like Herb (Sclerotium Poriae Cocoris). Many English translators have rendered this as latent pathogen. However, latent implies something lying inactive and this is not necessarily the case with viral *Fu Wen Xie*. These pathogens may be hidden and relatively asymptomatic, but Western medicine suggests that they are not always truly latent or inactive. Rather, they begin their disease process on the Inside and it takes time before this process become obvious on the Outside.

For instance, patients infected with HIV may be relatively symptom free but their T cell count may be plummeting as their immune system is plundered. Likewise, HSV, both I and II, may cause occult injury resulting in trigeminal neuralgia and sciatica without breaking out into obvious skin lesions. In the same way, HPV may be at work in the cervix where it causes dysplasia while the person may be relatively sign and symptom free were it not for the Pap smear. Therefore, although some degree of latency is implied in the Chinese concept of *Fu Xie*, I think retaining the more literal translation of Hidden Evil tallies better with our modern, clinical understanding of the danger of these pathogens.

The fact is, *Fu Xie* or Hidden Evils may be either Hidden and latent or Hidden but nonetheless active pathologically. Therefore, I have chosen to use the term Hidden Evils when translating the Chinese *Fu Xie* as a TCM concept. But, on occasion below, I will also sometimes refer to these pathogens' latency. In Western medicine, I believe the consensus is arising that HPV viruses may be maintained in a harmless latent state as long as the immune system is working properly. Unfortunately, everyone's immune system becomes deficient with age.

THE WESTERN IMMUNE SYSTEM & TCM

Previously I have written that there is no identical concept in TCM to the Western medical immune system.[15] This was specifically in response to some of my peers' simplistically equating the *Wei Qi* with the immune system. Based on the above Western description of HPV infection, it is clear that the Western immune system, both humoral and cellular, is involved in regressing HPV pathology, maintaining HPV in latency, and in defending from re-infection. Therefore, some further discussion of this issue is necessary.

Wei Qi, Defensive Qi, has its specific definition in TCM. It defends the Surface and warms the Interior, it circulates outside the *Jing Luo*, and it opens and closes the *Qi Men* or Gates of Qi. These are the pores, also called the *Gui Men* or the Evil Spirit Gates. *Wei Qi* is part of the Postnatal Qi in general. This Postnatal Qi may be referred to as the *Yuan Qi* or Original Qi, as Li Dong-yuan did, when meaning the total, undifferentiated Postnatal Qi. This *Yuan* is a different character from *Yuan* Source Qi which is the Prenatal Qi of the Kidneys. *Yuan* Original Qi may also be called the *Zhen Qi* or True Qi. However, in relation to pathogenic or Evil Qi, *Xie Qi*, it is referred to as *Zheng Qi* or Righteous Qi.

If there is any analogous concept in TCM to the immune system, it must simply be this *Zheng Qi*. *Zheng Qi* always implies its antagonistic relationship to *Xie Qi*. *Zheng Qi* is what maintains and restores health and what struggles with any Evil Qi. Beyond that, I do not think we should identify any other, more specific Qi with the immune system. Qi itself in its TCM functional definition contains the notion of defense from pathogenicity. There are five functions of the Qi according to TCM. These are to warm (*Wen*), defend (*Wei*), transport (*Yun*), transform (*Hua*), and to hold or consolidate (*Gu*).

However, from the perspective of the *San Bao* or Three Treasures, the basis of the Qi is the *Jing*. *Jing* Essence gives rise to the Qi and Qi gives rise to the *Shen* or Spirit. As Westerners, we tend to apply Western dichotomies and definitions to Chinese terms and concepts. Qi is often translated as energy and *Jing* as essential or fundamental substance. To the Western mind, this implies the old energy/matter dichotomy or dualism. However, the *Jing* itself is part of the *Zheng Qi*, and Qi sometimes is used in Chinese to describe what Westerners would consider matter. This is why some scholars, such as Paul U. Unschuld, refuse to accept the common Western TCM translation of Qi as energy. Unschuld, for instance, chooses to render this fundamental concept as influence.[16] Lu and Needham chose not to translate Qi at all except in a few instances where they use the Greek term *pneuma*.[17] As Nathan Sivin states, "Before modern times (i.e. influence from Western science) there was no separate conception of energy (as distinct from matter) in Chinese thought."[18] (Italics mine)

In any case, as we have seen above, *Jing* plays an important role in maintaining a Hidden Evil in latency. It is interesting to note that there is a statistical increase in HPV in the genital tracts of women after 50 and in men after 70.[19] Although it is believed that most men and women contract HPV in their second and third decades, the results of HPV infection often do not become obvious until much later. This tallies almost exactly with the statement in the *Nei Jing* that the *Jing* becomes Deficient at 7x7 or 49 in women and at 8x8 or 64 in men. This underscores the foundational role of the Kidneys in the creation of *Zheng Qi*. And, as we will see below, Kidney Yang and *Wei Qi* production are intimately related to the Large Intestine through the Internal Gate of the Triple Heater. Nevertheless, I do not believe TCM practitioners should equate the Western immune system with anything more specific than the *Zheng Qi* as long as we maintain a complete understanding of what the *Zheng Qi* is and where it comes from.

Adequate amounts of *Yuan* Original Qi are made as long as ascension of the Clear and descension of the Turbid proceed in a free-flowing and balanced fashion. Therefore, systemic balance is the *sine qua non* of insuring sufficient *Zheng Qi*. According to TCM theory, all the *Zang* and *Fu* are interdependent and mutually co-productive. When the *Zang Fu* function harmoniously, Qi and Blood are produced in abundance. From a Western medical point of view, this translates as immune competence. It is TCM diagnosis by *Bian Zheng* which allows for a precise, individualized description of how a particular patient's organism is out of balance. *Bian Zheng* diagnosis sees both the whole and the individual parts' relationship to that whole. Furthermore, treatment given based on such *Bian Zheng* diagnosis is effective for restoring functional balance and for optimizing the production of *Zheng Qi*.

THE TCM *BIAN ZHENG* OF CERVICAL CANCER

As mentioned above, there does exist in the English language literature the TCM *Bian Zheng* of cervical cancer. Since cervical dysplasia and cervical cancer, in fact, are a single disease continuum, TCM descriptions of the *Bian Zheng* diagnosis of cervical cancer are germane to dysplasia as well. A *Zheng* is the Pattern of a disease's manifestation. This Pattern describes the imbalance in body functions caused by the *Bing Yin* or etiological factors. Zhang Dai-zhao gives the following *Zheng* or Patterns describing most individuals with cervical cancer.[20]

Stagnant Toxins

The signs and symptoms of Stagnant Toxins in cervical cancer are profuse leukorrhea like rice-washing water (i.e. turbid) with offensive smell, distended pain of the lower abdomen, dry stools, yellow urine, a dark purple tongue with a sticky, white or sticky, yellow coating, and a slippery, rapid pulse. These signs and symptoms are often seen in patients with cauliflower (i.e. papilliform) or cavernous lesions.

Liver Blood/Kidney Yin Deficiency

The signs and symptoms of Liver Blood/Kidney Yin Deficiency cervical cancer are a bloody discharge, dizziness, tinnitus, knee and lumbar soreness and pain, a red tongue with scant or no coating, and a deep, thready pulse. These signs an symptoms are often seen in early stage or ulcerous conditions.

Qi Stagnation/Liver Depression (i.e. Depressive Heat)

The signs and symptoms of this *Zheng* as it manifests in relationship to cervical cancer are excessive leukorrhea, distention and fullness of the chest and costal regions, distended pain in the lower abdomen, bitter taste, sore throat, poor appetite, melancholy, emotional irritability, a normal tongue coating, and a wiry pulse. These signs and symptoms are often seen in nodular and ulcerous conditions.

Heart Blood/Spleen Qi Deficiency

This *Zheng* is characterized by continuous vaginal hemorrhage, excessive, dilute, white leukorrhea, palpitations, shortness of breath, dizziness, poor appetite, insomnia, frequent dreams, lumbar soreness, a normal tongue coating but fluted tongue body, and a deep, thready pulse. These signs and symptoms are often seen in cavernous and late stage conditions.

In addition, Hong-yen Hsu cites *Lectures on Surgery in Chinese Medicine* as including Spleen/Kidney Dual Deficiency instead of Heart/Spleen Dual Deficiency.[21]

Spleen/Kidney Dual Deficiency

The signs and symptoms of this *Zheng* are mental languor, lassitude, lumbago, backache, chest distention, profuse leukorrhea, muddy stools, a pale tongue with a normal coating, and a small, weak pulse.

Although these Patterns or *Zheng* are described as pure categories for didactic purposes, their signs and symptoms may vary within certain, professionally agreed upon boundaries. They are usually only the building blocks of an individualized diagnosis, and in their simple form, rarely adequately cover the idiosyncrasies of real-life patients. Therefore, it is not uncommon to find complex TCM diagnoses such as Liver Qi Stagnation leading to Depressive Heat complicated by Dampness and Heat and Stagnant Blood accumulated in the Lower Burner giving rise to PMS, *Yue Jing Xian Qi* (Menstruation Ahead of Schedule), and *Dai Xia* all in the same patient. The elements of such a complex diagnosis may change over time, with the phases of the moon, diet, menstrual cycle, External Invasions, emotional stress, exercise and activity, thus requiring constant adjustment and up-dating of the treatment.

In my clinical experience, most of the women I have treated for cervical dysplasia have some combination of Liver Qi/Liver Heat, Spleen Qi Deficiency, Heart Blood Deficiency, and Damp Heat and Stagnant Blood in the Lower Burner. This then is complicated by the venereally transmitted *Wen Fu Xie* or HPV. When this Hidden Evil becomes active, we must also say that it gives rise to Hot or Damp Hot Toxins.

Toxins are a somewhat difficult concept in Chinese medicine. They are called *Du* in Chinese which literally means poison but also has the connotation of malicious, cruel, or fierce. Toxins in Chinese medicine are not a general term for any pathogen similar to this term's use in Western naturopathy. Toxicity in that sense is covered by the more general term *Xie Qi* or Evil Qi. Rather, *Du* or Toxins describes a particularly virulent pathological condition most often associated with Dampness and/or Heat or Fire. In TCM, we can talk about Damp Toxins, Damp Heat Toxins, Hot Toxins, and Fire Toxins.

Modern TCM in general posits the existence of Toxins in essentially all cancers. This is because of cancer's special malignancy and rapid progress and also because, if left untreated, most cancers will develop into open lesions and abscesses which are described as Toxic in TCM. This latter fact is why much information about cancer is found in *Wai Ke* or External Medicine texts (incorrectly translated as surgery). Cancers being labelled Toxic is also because most cancers require special medicinals for their treatment. These special medicinals tend to have the ability to dissolve Toxins (*Jie Du*) appended to their other functions listed in *Ben Cao*. To a large extent, these *Jie Du* medicinals comprise the cancer-combatting or *Kang Ai* category of TCM medicinals.

It is extremely important for practitioners to remember that the *Zheng* is not the cause of the disease. The cause of the disease is the *Bing Yin*. The *Zheng* is the description of the manifestation of the disease and the patient's overall, individual condition. It is the *Zheng* which individualizes the patient's diagnosis and, therefore, their subsequent treatment. It is diagnosis by *Bian Zheng* which allows TCM to treat the whole person as opposed to some abstract concept of disease. However, for this to happen, the individual diagnosis by *Bian Zheng* must be individually tailored. The patient should not be made to fit into a textbook *Zheng*, but rather, a complicated *Zheng* should be elaborated to adequately cover the entirety of an individual's signs and symptoms. For further advice on how to tailor individual diagnoses by *Bian Zheng*, see my *Sticking to the Point, A Rational Methodology for the Step by Step Formulation & Administration of an Acupuncture Treatment*.[22]

CHAPTER THREE
THE REMEDIAL TCM TREATMENT OF CERVICAL INTRAEPITHELIAL NEOPLASIA

Although Chinese medicine says that the Superior Physician prevents the arisal of disease, most American women seek treatment only after receiving a bad or positive Pap. Therefore, we will discuss cervical dysplasia's remedial treatment first and secondarily its prevention from recurrence. My remedial TCM treatment of cervical dysplasia is logically derived from the above TCM discussion of CIN, its Western and Chinese etiologies, and its diagnosis by *Bian Bing* and *Bian Zheng*. For me, a comprehensive treatment plan means adjusting my patient's diet, exercise, and life-style in addition to prescribing internal medicines and performing external therapies. Further, we must also say something about sex during the course of remedial treatment and the treatment of concurrent, complicating conditions, such as candidiasis.

DIET

Although each patient's dietary therapy should be prescribed based on their individual *Zheng*, still, in general, the following guidelines are what I tend to repeat to my patients with CIN.

1) One should eat as few Damp foods as possible, including

sugar and sweets; oils, greases, fried, and fatty foods; cold and excessive liquids with meals; raw fruits and vegetables and especially citrus fruits, pineapples, and raw tomatoes; dairy products; nuts; and alcohol. Since ice cream is Sweet, Cold, and Damp, it is an especially dangerous food for persons attempting to limit or dispel Dampness within.

It is the Spleen which is primarily in charge of transporting and transforming Liquids. Since Dampness especially distresses the Spleen, avoiding Damp foods benefits the Spleen. According to TCM theory, a strong Spleen can keep the Liver in check by way of the Five Phase *Ke* cycle, and strengthening the Spleen is considered the first way to treat an aberrant Liver. Therefore, avoiding Damp foods not only minimizes the production of Internal Dampness but also checks an Excessive Liver. Since CIN in American women is almost always associated with some amount of Liver Qi, avoiding Damp foods serves a dual purpose.

2) One should eat as little Hot, Acrid, spicy food as possible. Although I find forbidding foods completely to my patients counterproductive, CIN patients generally should not eat any Hot, Acrid, spicy foods at all. Spicy foods are addicting and they have become an increasingly popular part of the American diet. Like smoking and alcohol, spicy foods do temporarily disperse Stagnant Liver Qi, but their net effect is to cause Internal Heat (*Nei Re*). They also waste both Lung Qi and Yin. Since Lung Qi is so important for checking and dispersing Liver Qi, maintenance of healthy Lung Qi is extremely important in the treatment of CIN. Alcohol is both Hot and Acrid as well as Damp.

3) One should avoid over-eating in general, eating too hurriedly, or eating under stress. All three of these tend to cause Food Stagnation. Food Stagnation is a common complicating factor in many person's TCM diagnosis. TCM

texts make Food Stagnation seem episodic and relatively inconsequential. However, Food Stagnation is mutually co-productive with Liver Qi Stagnation. Food Stagnation tends to aggravate accumulation of Phlegm and Dampness. In addition, when Food Stagnation persists over time, the Stomach becomes Hot. Heat in the Stomach is co-productive with Liver Heat and such Transformative Heat, especially in the Liver, needs to be avoided in CIN patients.

Cervical dysplasia patients should be counselled to eat a low fat, relatively bland diet emphasizing freshly cooked vegetables and complex carbohydrates. This is similar to the Pritikin and Macrobiotic diets. For further information on Chinese dietary therapy, see my and Honora Lee Wolfe's *Prince Wen Hui's Cook*[1] and my *Nine Ounces, A Nine Part Program for The Prevention of AIDS in HIV Positive Persons*.[2]

EXERCISE

Remedial exercise for CIN patients can be divided into 2 types: general aerobic exercise and specifically pelvic, remedial exercise.

1) Aerobic Exercise

Women in their 20s, 30s, and early 40s with CIN should be counselled to get regular *aerobic* exercise. The definition of aerobic exercise is any activity which raises the pulse 80% over its resting rate and keeps it there a continuous twenty minutes. This should be repeated not less than every 48 hours, being sure not to let a maximum of 72 hours elapse between exercise sessions.

Aerobic exercise mobilizes the Qi and Blood. Therefore, it dissipates Stagnation of the Qi, Blood, Dampness, Phlegm,

Food, and Heat. After 3 months of regular aerobic exercise, a patient's appetite, energy, mood, sleep, digestion, elimination, and warmth in their extremities will all have improved markedly.

In particular, many women with Liver Qi experience cold hands and feet. This is called *Si Ni* or the Four Counterflows. The Qi which should be dispersed to the extremities implodes inward. This creates False Cold signs and symptoms on the Outside with True Heat Internally. This is corroborated by a patient's rapid, wiry pulse and reddish *Qing* or purplish tongue. Aerobic exercise reverses this implosion and disperses the Internal Heat outwards. Promotion of diaphoresis is an accepted treatment for Internal Heat if there is no sweating.

2) Remedial Exercise for the Pelvis

Besides regular aerobic exercise, there are two other systems of remedial exercise which can be useful adjuncts to the remedial treatment of CIN in particular and of menopathies in general. As discussed above, a large part of the TCM treatment plan I am advancing has to do with changing the internal environment of the pelvis. Stagnation of Qi and Blood in the pelvis tends to engender Evil Heat and the accumulation of pathologic Dampness. Such a Damp, Hot, Stagnant environment is the perfect milieu for the flourishing of *Wen Re* or Warm Hot Evils. Such an environment can be changed by remedial pelvic exercise.

Ludmila Mojzis, a Czechoslovakian physical therapist, 20 years ago created a system of exercises meant to correct faulty body posture; relieve visible and palpable spasms along the lumbar spine, spasms of the inner thigh, and spasms of the muscles attached to the coccyx; and to strengthen weakened, hypotonic buttock and abdominal muscles. Women with infertility and other menstrual and reproductive tract problems doing these exercises have reported normalization of their menstrual cycles and increased fertility. Over the last 20 years, literally thousands of women with menstrual and reproductive problems have been treated successfully by this system of exercise. In particular, the women whom Mojzis singles out as the most responsive to her system of remedial exercise are those with dysmenorrhea and dyspareunia or pain with intercourse. These women would likely be diagnosed as suffering from endometriosis by Western medicine and in Chinese medicine usually suffer from Stagnant Qi and Blood.

By correcting posture, strengthening and exercising the intrinsic and extrinsic muscles of the pelvic girdle, and by relieving muscular spasm, the Mojzis Method activates and regulates the flow of Qi and Blood in the Lower Burner. It is also interesting to note that Vaclav Hlavaty, MD in his preface to *Children of Your Own: The Mojzis Method*, says that considerable improvement of the pelvic environment can be achieved in from 3-6 months using this method.[3] This is the same period of time I have found generally necessary for the successful treatment of most menopathies using TCM. As an ex-*Tai Ji* and *Qi Gong* instructor, I am well aware of the healing benefits of correcting body posture, releasing chronic muscular spasm, and promoting a more healthful, free-flowing use of the body.

Another, somewhat similar method of remedial exercise which concentrates on the muscles of the lower abdomen and pelvic girdle is the Pilates Method. Joseph Pilates was a German osteopath, gymnast, and boxer active during the first half of this century. In describing the essence of a Pilates movement, Romana Kryzanwska, a long-time student and now Pilates teacher, frequently speaks of "flowing motion outward from a strong center." This center is the *Qi Hai/Dan Tian*. Pilates also believed in getting the blood pumping and breathing both correctly and fully, thus, in essence, promoting the free flow of

Qi and Blood.

Both the Mojzis and Pilates Methods are taught in the United States. Both systems can be useful adjuncts to the TCM treatment of CIN and various menopathies. Women with sedentary jobs, low back pain, dysmenorrhea, and flaccid abdomens are especially good candidates for either of these methods. Other remedial exercise systems, such as Hatha yoga and Feldenkrais floor work, may also be tailored to achieve the same results, and even belly dancing may be equally as effective. For further information on the Mojzis Method, see *Children of Your Own: The Mojzis Method* written by Ludmila Mojzis.

DEEP RELAXATION

Deep relaxation is the single best way to treat Liver Qi due to stress and emotional upset. By this I mean both somatic as well as psychic deep relaxation. This allows the *Jin* Sinews to relax thus facilitating relaxation of the Liver. The Qi then regulates itself and harmony is automatically restored. In addition, deep relaxation calms the *Shen*. This likewise has a systemic regularizing, harmonizing effect on the entire organism.

I typically write my CIN patients a prescription for deep relaxation. I require them to do a progressive, guided, deep relaxation tape every single day for 100 consecutive days. Such tapes begin with the patient lying down on their back and then guide the patient's will and awareness to relax their entire musculature and physical being beginning from the head and ending at the feet. At the end of 100 hundred days, the patient will register definite improvement in their appetite, digestion, elimination, energy, mood, sleep, and warmth in their extremities. In addition, such guided, progressive, daily, deep relaxation will train the patient how to release pent-up Qi during their daily life quicker and more effectively. However, for these therapeutic results to be accomplished, this deep relaxation must be practiced daily. It must become a part of each and every of the patient's days.

Aerobic exercise and deep relaxation used in tandem are extremely effective for regulating the Qi and clearing Internal Heat. Exercise dissipates already accumulated Heat, and deep relaxation prevents it from accumulating in the first place. In our clinic, we call diet, exercise, and deep relaxation the Three Free Therapies. Not only do they not cost the patient anything, they are the foundation for comprehensive healing and preventive maintenance. I try to make it as clear as possible to my patients that diet, exercise, and deep relaxation are the foundation of their cure and that any other professional therapies over and above these are adjuncts to this threefold, basic regime.

HERBAL MEDICINE

I divide herbal medicine for cervical dysplasia into internally and externally administered remedies. It is my experience that the quickest and best results come from a co-ordinated use of both.

INTERNAL REMEDIES

For the first 3 menstrual cycles after commencing TCM therapy for CIN, I usually prescribe herbal medicine as individually tailored decoctions. Although this book is not a text on *Fang Ji Xue* or the study of writing prescriptions, TCM methodology is based on first picking a guiding formula professionally agreed upon corresponding to both the diagnosis by *Bian Bing* and *Bian Zheng*. This then is modified by deleting unnecessary ingredients not germane to the patient's particular signs and symptoms and adding other ingredients necessary to address either complications in the *Ben* Root or *Biao* Branch.

I begin with the patient's TCM *Bian Bing* diagnosis, remembering that CIN is not a Chinese *Bing* or disease category. Therefore, I first identify the patient's Chinese *Fu Ke* or gynecological category. For a discussion of these *Fu Ke* categories, see *A Handbook of Traditional Chinese Gynecology.*[4] In my experience, the most common Chinese disease categories with which my dysplasia patients present are *Yue Jing Xian Qi* (Menstruation Ahead of Schedule), *Tong Jing* (Painful Menstruation), *Jing Xing Ru Fang Zhang Tong* (Premenstrual Breast Distention & Pain), *Dai Xia* (Abnormal Vaginal Discharge), and *Yin Chuang* (Vaginal Lesions).

Next, I try to determine the *Bing Yin* or etiologies of the patient's disease and its *Bing Ji* or disease mechanism. This is followed by a TCM diagnosis by *Bian Zheng*, remembering that, in most cases, the Pattern described will be a complex scenario made up of two or more simple, textbook *Zheng*. A guiding prescription is selected based on both the *Bing* and the *Zheng*, which is then modified to meet the individual patient's needs. If there is any vaginal infection characterized by either *Dai Xia* or genital lesions accompanied by erythema and pain, these should be treated first as an acute *Biao* or Branch condition. If there is no obvious acute vaginal infection, I recommend addressing any Chinese menopathy present, such as Painful Menstruation, Premenstrual Breast Distention (and PMS in general), and/or Menstruation Ahead of Schedule.

Treatment of any of these Chinese disease states will necessarily restore balance and harmony to the internal environment of the organism in general and of the pelvis in particular. In most cases, menopathies should only require 3-4 cycles to treat with marked or complete improvement. Repeat Pap smears should not be performed until any obvious Chinese disease states have been cured or substantially ameliorated because, until or unless these are eliminated, it is improbable that a negative Pap will be obtained. Regulation of the menstrual cycle implies regulation of the hormones. Since hormones play such a large part in mediating the immune response, balancing these hormones likewise benefits the competence of the immune system.

Although there are a number of guiding prescriptions from which one might chose based on the range of Chinese disease categories and *Zheng* which individual patients may present, there are several guiding formulas I would like to discuss since I find I use these in the majority of my CIN patients.

Xiao Yao San (Free & Easy Powder, aka Rambling Powder)

This is one of the most commonly used gynecological formulas in the TCM repertoire. It treats a wide range of Chinese disease categories when their *Bian Zheng* diagnosis is Liver Qi, Blood Deficiency, and Spleen Deficiency with some element of Dampness. Its standard ingredients are:

    Radix Bupleuri
    Radix Angelicae Sinensis
    Radix Paeoniae Albae
    Rhizoma Atractylodis Macrocephalae
    Sclerotium Poriae Cocoris
    Herba Menthae
    Radix Praeparatus Glycyrrhizae
    Rhizoma Recens Zingiberis

In this formula, Bupleurum is meant to dredge the Liver, regulate the Qi, and relieve constraint. Peony and Dang Gui nourish the Blood and relax the Liver. In tandem with

Bupleurum, these three ingredients regulate the *Chong* and *Ren*. Atractylodes and Poria tonify the Spleen and benefit the Qi at the same time as eliminating Dampness both through transformation and transportation. In combination with Bupleurum, these three ingredients harmonize Liver Wood and Spleen Earth. In addition, Poria helps to calm the Heart Spirit. Fieldmint (Herba Menthae) helps to dredge the Liver and dissipate constrained Qi. At the same time, it also clears low to moderate levels of Liver/Stomach Heat. Honey-baked Licorice tonifies the Spleen and benefits the Qi while also promoting Stomach Fluids so as to protect from Bupleurum's tendency to plunder Yin. Further, Licorice tonifies Heart Qi thus benefitting the *Shen* and, therefore, the entire organism. Fresh Ginger harmonizes the Stomach and helps eliminate Dampness. Since Dang Gui is a greasy ingredient, it aids in that ingredient's digestibility.

Xiao Yao San can be modified in a myriad of ways. Since Liver/Spleen and Qi and Blood disharmonies are so common, it is no wonder that this is one of TCM's most famous and often used formulas. Dr. C.S. Cheung, in *On Prescription, Vol. 2*, lists a large number of modifications of this basic formula.[5] However, there is one modification which is pre-eminently important. This is called in Chinese Dan Zhi Xiao Yao San (Moutan & Gardenia Free & Easy Powder). Its ingredients are:

    Radix Bupleuri
    Radix Angelicae Sinensis
    Radix Paeoniae Albae
    Cortex Radicis Moutan
    Fructus Gardeniae
    Rhizoma Atractylodis Macrocephalae
    Sclerotium Poriae Cocoris
    Radix Praeparatus Glycyrrhizae

Some TCM texts list Fieldmint and Ginger as standard ingredients of this prescription and other says that, when Moutan and Gardenia are added, these are routinely deleted. Be that as it may, the addition of Moutan and Gardenia changes the basic *Zheng* for which this formula is prescribed. Although the formula still tonifies the Spleen, eliminates Dampness, and nourishes the Blood, this modification is specifically indicated for clearing Depressive Liver Heat. This formula can be further modified to treat Menstruation Ahead of Schedule due to Depressive Heat, the most common variety of early period; *Dai Xia* due to Damp Heat when the Heat is derived from a depressed Liver; Painful Menstruation due to Mutual Entanglement of Stagnant Qi, Depressive Heat, and Damp Heat in the Lower Burner; and Premenstrual Breast Distention complicated by Depressive Liver Heat.

Another modification of Xiao Yao San is to alternate Dan Zhi Xiao Yao San with Gui Pi Tang (Return the Spleen Decoction) with the addition of Bupleurum. This combination is indicated for the treatment of Liver/Spleen Disharmony with Qi and Blood Deficiency and Stagnation of Damp Heat in the Lower Burner. It can be used by women with gynecological neoplasms or by men with testicular and prostate problems. Gui Pi Tang in TCM is specifically indicated for the treatment of Heart Blood/Spleen Qi Deficiency. However, when combined with Dan Zhi Xiao Yao San, it skillfully addresses a more complicated and commonly encountered scenario. In this case, there is Liver Qi and, therefore, Blood Stagnation below entangled with Damp Heat. Dampness percolates down from the Middle because of insufficient Spleen Qi to transport and transform Liquids. This Spleen Qi Deficiency incapacitates the Spleen from sending up the Pure part of the Fluids to be transformed into Blood in the Heart. This then leaves the Heart Blood insufficient to nourish and secure the *Shen*. Liver Heat, however, does ascend into the Upper Burner tending to agitate the Heart. Therefore, there is a mixture of Liver

Heat/Heart Blood Insufficiency signs and symptoms, including palpitations and irritability.

When this regime is used, Gui Pi Tang with Bupleurum (Gui Pi Tang Jia Chai Hu) is taken in the morning and the Dan Zhi Xiao Yao San is taken at night. Xiao Yao San, Dan Zhi Xiao Yao San, and Gui Pi Tang are all obtainable as desiccated extracts from Qualiherbs in Santa Fe Springs, CA. Qualiherbs also supplies desiccated extracts of individual herbs, such as Bupleurum, which can then be easily added to the powdered formula. Of course, if herbs are taken as a freshly decocted, bulk-dispensed prescription, the practitioner is free to modify the formula in any way which seems appropriate. However, when two separate formulas are used in the same day, this is not so easy to manage either time or cost-wise. The ingredients in Gui Pi Tang are:

        Radix Panacis Ginseng Seu Codonopsis Pilosulae
        Radix Astragali Seu Hedysari
        Radix Angelicae Sinensis
        Fructus Aridus Euphorbiae Longanae
        Rhizoma Atractylodis Macrocephalae
        Radix Saussureae Seu Vladimiriae
        Sclerotium Poriae Cocoris
        Radix Polygalae Tenuifoliae
        Fructus Zizyphi Jujubae
        Semen Zizyphi Spinosae
        Radix Praeparatus Glycyrrhizae
        Rhizoma Recens Zingiberis

Taiwanese Empirical Formula for the Treatment of Cervical Cancer

In *Treating Cancer with Chinese Herbs*, Hong-yen Hsu gives a formula for the treatment of uterine/cervical cancer developed by a Chinese medical college in Taiwan.[6] The ingredients in this formula are:

> Radix Scutellariae Barbatae
> Herba Solani Lyrati
> Herba Cum Radice Taraxaci Mongolici
> Radix Angelicae Sinensis
> Radix Paeoniae Albae
> Rhizoma Atractylodis Macrocephalae
> Sclerotium Poriae Cocoris
> Pericarpium Citri Reticulatae Viride
> Radix Bupleuri
> Radix Salviae Miltorrhizae

Following this basic formula, a list of additions are given for different presenting symptoms and complicating *Zheng*. However, it is obvious that this formula is itself a modification of Xiao Yao San. Scutellaria Barbata, Solanum Lyratum, and Taraxicum are all ingredients from the *Kang Ai* or cancer-combatting category of TCM medicinals. These ingredients all clear Heat and dissolve Toxins. In addition, Scutellaria Barbata facilitates Water, relieves swelling, and disperses Stagnant Blood. Solanum Lyratum also facilitates Water, relieves swelling, and is empirically specific for the treatment of cervical cancer. And Taraxicum, aka Dandelion, dissolves Fire Toxins, disperses Nodulations, and has a special tropism for the breasts. Green Citrus Peel aids Bupleurum in dredging the Liver and regulating the Qi. It cracks more serious Qi Stagnation and reduces Accumulations. It also dries Dampness and transforms Phlegm. Salvia invigorates the Blood and breaks up Stagnant Blood. It also clears Heat and soothes irritability. Some practitioners believe Salvia to have within itself all the properties of the four ingredients of Si Wu Tang (Four Ingredient Decoction: Radix Rehmanniae Seu Rehmanniae Conquitae, Radix Angelicae Sinensis, Radix Paeoniae Albae Seu Rubrae, & Radix Ligustici Chuanxiong).

This modification of Xiao Yao San is significant in that it incorporates *Qu Xie* or attacking Evil ingredients specific for clearing Heat and dissolving Toxins and also combatting cancer. Because the etiology of CIN is, in part, a Warm Hidden, Pestilential Evil, the addition of Heat-clearing, Toxin-dissolving, cancer-combatting ingredients makes sense. For the last year, I have been judiciously incorporating such ingredients into my treatment of dysplasia with good results.

The following is a list of TCM *Kang Ai* medicinals which I select from when modifying formulas for my dysplasia patients. These should not be added indiscriminately but based on an assessment of both *Ben* and *Biao*. For instance, if there are painful, fibrocystic breasts, the inclusion of Taraxicum makes sense. Whereas, if there is Yellow *Dai*, Cortex Ailanthi Altissimae is especially appropriate since it is empirically specific for the treatment of cervical dysplasia and *Dai Xia*. If there is Painful Menstruation with Mutual Entanglement of Stagnation with Damp Heat, Radix Patriniae Heterophyllae is especially effective. And, when there is Excessive Menstruation (*Yue Jing Guo Duo*, i.e. menorrhagia) with Depressive Heat and Stagnant Blood, Herba Selaginellae Doerderleinii is particularly useful.

Kang Ai Medicinals for the Treatment of CIN

Rhizoma Paridis Polyphyllae is Bitter, slightly Cold, mildly Toxic, and enters the Liver Channel. It clears Heat, dissolves Toxins, reduces swelling, extinguishes Wind, stops pain, and suppresses convulsions.

Fructus Bruceae Javanicae is Bitter and Cold and enters the Large Intestine Channel. It dissolves Toxins, relieves swelling, dries Dampness, kills Worms, and is a specific against papilloma virus. It is also used for chronic dysentery-like disorders which wax and wane and alternating hard and soft stools. It should be used with care with a weak Stomach/Spleen and is often combined with Fructus Aridus Euphorbiae Longanae.

Herba Crotolariae Sessiliflorae is Bitter, Bland, and Neutral although some sources say it is Sweet and Warm. It clears Heat and dissolves Toxins, combats cancer, and is a specific for skin and cervical cancers.

Radix Patriniae Heterophyllae is Bitter, Sour, Astringent, and Cold and enters the Liver Channel. It clears Heat, dissolves Toxins, dries Dampness, stops bleeding, stops *Dai Xia*, and is a specific for cervical and liver cancers. It is good for dysmenorrhea accompanied by an early period and/or breakthrough bleeding due to Mutual Entanglement of Damp Heat and Stagnant Qi and Blood.

Herba Scutellariae Barbatae is Acrid and Cool or Cold. It enters the Heart and Lungs. It clears Heat, dissolves Toxins, facilitates Water, relieves swelling, disperses Stagnant Blood, combats cancer, and is a common *Qing Re, Jie Du* ingredient.

Herba Cum Radice Taraxici Mongolici is Sweet, Bitter, and Cold and enters the Liver and Stomach. It clears Heat and dissolves Fire Toxins, disperses Nodulations, relieves swelling, promotes lactation, and has a special tropism for the chest. It is used for breast, lung, and thyroid cancers. It should be included especially if there are fibrocystic breasts and premenstrual breast and/or nipple pain.

Herba Solani Lyrati is Bitter, slightly Cold, and enters the Liver and Stomach. It clears Heat and dissolves Toxins, facilitates Water, relieves swelling, and combats cancer. It is a specific for liver, stomach, lung, bladder, and uterine and cervical cancers.

Cortex Ailanthi Altissimae is Bitter, Astringent, and Cold and enters the Stomach and Large Intestine Channels. It clears Heat, dries Dampness, stops diarrhea, stops bleeding, stops *Dai Xia*, and is a specific for cervical and intestinal cancers.

Folium Cycasis Revolutae is Sweet and slightly Warm and enters the Stomach Channel. It activates the Blood, relieves swelling, transforms Phlegm, eliminates Dampness, and combats cancer. It is a specific for lung, stomach, liver, uterine, cervical, and mesopharangeal cancers.

Herba Selaginellae Doerderleinii clears Heat and dissolves Toxins. It cools the Blood, stops bleeding, dispels Stagnant Blood, and activates the Blood.

Rhizoma Smilacis Glabrae is Sweet, Sour, and Neutral and enters the Liver and Stomach Channels. It dissolves Damp Heat Toxins, eliminates swelling, activates the Blood, expels Wind, clears and eliminates Damp Heat from the skin, and is especially useful for Damp Heat Toxins in the genitalia.

Fructus Broussonetiae is Sweet and Cold and enters the Liver, Spleen, and Kidneys. It nourishes the Kidneys, clears the Liver, facilitates Water, benefits urination, and is used for debility of the loins, edema, abdominal distention, and Blood Deficiency.

Spica Prunella Vulgaris is Sweet, Acrid, slightly Bitter, and Cold and enters the Liver, Gallbladder, and Lung Channels. It clears Liver Fire, brightens the eyes, clears Heat, dissipates Nodulations, disperses Stagnations and Accumulations, and is specifically used if there is lymph node enlargement including those of the groin.

Pulvis Indigo Naturalis is Salty and Cold and enters the Liver and Lung Channels. It clears Heat and dissolves Toxins, disperses Stagnant Fire by purging the Liver, combats cancer, and is anti-viral.

Radix Sophorae Flavescentis is Sweet, Bitter, and Warm and enters the Heart, Liver, Stomach, Small Intestine, and Large Intestine Channels. It clears Heat and dissolves Toxins, kills Worms, facilitates Water, benefits urination, disperses Wind and stops itching, clears and eliminates Damp Heat from the Lower Burner and skin, and is a specific for cervical, liver, large intestine, and skin cancer.

Rhizoma Zedoariae is Sweet, Bitter, and Warm and enters the Liver and Spleen Channels. It softens the Hard, disperses Nodulations, cracks Stasis, and activates the Qi. It is a specific for uterine and cervical cancers accompanied by Substantial Stagnant Blood.

Rhizoma Arisaematis is Bitter, Warm, and Toxic and enters the Lung, Liver, and Spleen Channels. It transforms Phlegm, disperses Nodulation, extinguishes Wind, and suppresses convulsions. It is a specific for lung, esophageal, and cervical cancers accompanied by Phlegm.

Semen Strychnotis is Sweet, Warm, and strongly Toxic. It enters the Liver and Spleen Channels. It searches Wind Toxins, disperses Nodulation, relieves swelling, activates the *Luo*, and stops pain. Do not exceed 1-1.5 g p.d. internally.

Lacca Sinica Exiccata, aka Resina Rhi Verniciferae, activates the Blood and disperses Stagnant Blood and Accumulations. It kills Worms and is used to treat amenorrhea and abdominal masses.

In addition, since *Fu Wen Xie* specifically reside in the *Xue Fen*, ingredients may also be profitably chosen from which treat that energetic phase. According to Wiseman and Ellis, compilers of *Fundamentals of Chinese Medicine*, there are two treatment methods for addressing *Wen Xie* in the *Xue Fen*. These are to *Liang Xue* or cool the Blood and to *Qing Xue* to clear (Heat) from the Blood. Dr. Liu, author of *The Essential Book of Traditional Chinese Medicine*, suggests this latter course in treating *Fu Wen Xie*.[8] Ingredients which specifically clear Heat from the Blood Phase include:

>   Radix Rehmanniae
>   Radix Scrophulariae
>   Radix Lithospermi Seu Arnebiae
>   Folium Isatidis
>   Radix Isatidis
>   Flos Lonicerae
>   Radix Paeoniae Rubrae
>   Cortex Radicis Moutan
>   Cornu Rhinoceri

Because this last ingredient is obtained from an endangered species, it should no longer be used in TCM except in extreme, life-threatening cases. Cornu Bubali (Shui Niu Jiao or Water Buffalo Horn) should be used instead due to the worldwide abundance of this product. When Cornu Bubali is substituted for Cornu Rhinoceri, its dosage is substantially increased. Subhuti Dharmananda questions the efficacy of both these horns and suggests that, in the treatment of viral problems, the above plant-derived medicinals should be used instead.[9]

Chai Hu Gui Zhi Tang (Bupleurum & Cinnamon Decoction)

When the Liver becomes Excess, it typically vents onto Earth. This not only causes Spleen Deficiency but also Heat and upward perversion of the Stomach. Heat can rise up the *Xu Li* from the Stomach to the Heart, thus transferring Heat to the Blood and thence back to the Liver and also disturbing the Heart *Shen*. In addition, Heat rising from the Liver and

Stomach tends to accumulate in the Lungs where it disturbs the Lungs' capacity to control the Liver and clear and descend the Qi. If there is Dampness in the Spleen, this may cause Phlegm being drafted up into the Lungs, neck, axillae, and breasts. If the Stomach, Liver, Heart, and Lungs all become overheated, the *Ming Men* in general tends to flare upwards, since the *Ming Men* is, in part, the Heat of these Organs. (See Appendix II for a fuller explanation of the *Ming Men vis a vis* the *Zang Fu*.) The *Ming Men* thus tends to lose its Root in the Kidneys, hence failing to energize and warm the flow of Qi and Blood in the Lower Burner. This is a common though complex Pattern found in many middle-aged Americans, both men and women, and it is remediable herbally by administering Chai Hu Gui Zhi Tang. The ingredients in this formula are:

    Radix Bupleuri
    Radix Panacis Ginseng Seu Codonopsis Pilosulae
    Radix Scutellaria Baicalensis
    Radix Paeoniae Albae
    Rhizoma Pinelliae
    Sclerotium Poriae Cocoris
    Ramulus Cinnamomi
    Radix Praeparatus Glycyrrhizae
    Fructus Zizyphi Jujubae
    Rhizoma Recens Zingiberis

In this formula, Bupleurum again dredges the Liver Qi, whereas Peony relaxes the Liver. Ginseng or Codonopsis tonify the Spleen. Pinellia eliminates Dampness, transforms Phlegm, harmonizes the Stomach, and descends the Lungs. Scutellaria clears Heat from the Lungs, Liver, and Stomach. Poria promotes urination and aids Pinellia in eliminating Dampness. It also aids Ginseng/Codonopsis in tonifying the Spleen. Cinnamon redirects Heat downwards from the Upper Burner and especially from the Heart to its Root in the Lower Burner and Kidneys. In addition, it dissipates outward Internal

Evil Heat imploded within. Licorice, Red Dates, and Ginger all help tonify the Spleen and Heart, harmonize the Stomach, and protect the Stomach against the drying effects of Bupleurum and Cinnamon. This formula can be used where there are signs of Internal Heat since it dissipates this Heat outward and returns *Ming Men Huo* to its Root, at the same time as clearing with Cold ingredients pathologic Heat from the Liver, Stomach, and Lungs.

Bupleurum and Cinnamon Decoction is a very well crafted formula which addresses a very commonly encountered, complex Pattern. It can be modified with additions and subtractions in order to make it even more specific for the treatment of various Branch symptoms accompanying the Root disharmony. For further insights into the complex Pattern which Chai Hu Gui Zhi Tang addresses, see my "Yin Yang and the Mechanisms of Internal Disease" in *Blue Poppy Essays 1988*.[10]

Ping Xiao Dan (Levelling & Dispersing Elixir)

Ping Xiao Dan is a formula created by Jia Kun, a famous TCM oncologist working in Xian in the People's Republic of China. This prescription is the basis for his treatment of cancer, giving it remedially at least during the initial stages of *all* malignancies.[11] The ingredients in this formula are:

> Fructus Immaturus Citri Seu Ponciri
> Tuber Curcumae
> Sal Nitri
> Lacca Sinica Exsiccata
> Alumen
> Semen Strychnotis
> Excrementum Trogopterori Seu Pteromi
> Herba Agrimoniae

Excrementum Trogopterori, Lacca Sinica, and Alumen disperse Stagnation, activate the Blood, clear Heat and eliminate Dampness. Sal Nitri clears Heat and refreshes the body Organs. Semen Strychnotis activates the *Luo*, transforms Phlegm, disperse Nodulations, and relieves swelling. And Herba Agrimoniae and Fructus Immaturus Citri Seu Ponciri combine to crack Stagnant Qi and reduce Accumulation, direct the Qi downward, and clear Dampness and Heat. As a whole, this formula attacks Evil in the form of Stagnant Qi, Blood, Heat, Dampness, Phlegm, and Food.

I sometimes add this powder to other formulas as if it were a single ingredient, in which case it is taken orally and washed down with the decoction. Usually I do this only at the beginning of a course of treatment and only in the week before the period. The recommended dosage is 1.5-6 grams TID. I use this formula if there is pronounced Qi and Blood Stagnation entangled with Damp Heat which has lingered for a long time and has caused Stagnation in the *Luo*. Because this formula was especially designed for treating malignancies by a TCM oncologist, its use helps to reassure patients nervous about cancer, whether they currently have cancer or are just afraid of developing it. As we will see below, it can be used both remedially and preventively. However, its use should be restricted to those patients with predominately Excess conditions or else should be administered in combination with tonics.

These several TCM formulas discussed above for internal administration are just the most common guiding prescriptions I tend to use. They are *not* categorical treatments for cervical dysplasia. It is important that the practitioner choose the right guiding prescription for an individual patient based on *Bian Bing* and *Bian Zheng* and then modify that prescription accordingly. The *Bing* or TCM disease states which I address first are Menstruation Ahead of Schedule or any other abnormal bleeding, Abnormal Vaginal Discharge, and/or PMS, which in TCM texts is discussed under Premenstrual Breast Distention. Practitioners will find further ideas about alternative guiding prescriptions for the various *Zheng* describing these disease states in TCM gynecology texts, such as *A Handbook of Traditional Chinese Gynecology*.[12]

EXTERNAL REMEDIES

There are a number of external or topical remedies which I find important in the comprehensive treatment of cervical dysplasia. These include cervical powders and suppositories, douches, abdominal compresses and plasters, and even enemas.

A) Cervical Powders

There are two cervical powders I commonly use in the treatment of CIN. These are applied to the cervix either by a intravaginal applicator or on the head of a tampon. They are usually applied before bed at night and kept in place till morning.

1) Yin Healing Powder

      Cinnabaris
      Borneolum
      Borax
      Pulvis Indigo

This powder is based on a Chinese formula to which I have added Pulvis Indigo. This formula clears Heat, dissolves Toxins, dries Dampness, prevents putrefaction, generates New Flesh, relieves swelling, dissipates Nodulations, combats cancer, and is anti-viral. Pulvis Indigo, made from Isatis Tinctorius, has demonstrated anti-viral activity *in vitro*. Since I believe that CIN is, in part, a viral infection, I have added this ingredient for that reason. In general, my patients like the cool, mentholated feeling of this powder. I use this powder when dysplasia is mild. It can be used throughout the cycle except during menstruation itself.

2) Qing Peng San (Borax & Alum Powder)

This is also a Chinese formula to which I have made an addition for the same reason as above. Its ingredients are:

> Pulvis Corticis Phellodendri
> Pulvis Radicis Lithospermi Seu Arnebiae
> Borax
> Alumen
> Borneolum
> Pulvis Indigo
> Pulvis Herbae Larreae

Qing Peng San is indicated for the adjunctive treatment of cervical dysplasia when there is more prominent Dampness and Heat. Besides possessing the same functions as Yin Healing Powder above, it also stops *Dai* or Abnormal Vaginal Discharge. The ingredient I have added is Larrea or Chaparral. Chaparral has well-known anti-viral activity and has long been used for the treatment of warts. Since cervical dysplasia is partly due to the genital wart virus, its inclusion seems logical to me.

B) Suppositories

There are a number of vaginal suppositories which can be used in the adjunctive treatment of CIN. They can be divided into three general categories: 1) those which are escarotic; 2) those which clear and eliminate Damp Heat; and 3) those which promote the generation of New Flesh.

Escarosis means the killing of the epithelial cells infected with the Hidden Evil Toxins or HPV and the sloughing or exfoliation of these dead cells. This is a species of *Qu Xie* or Evil-attacking therapy. I use such escarotic therapy when CIN is more severe or persistent. It is usually not necessary for the treatment of mild dysplasia but is definitely recommended for the treatment of severe dysplasia and CIS.

Because this is a *Qu Xie* therapy, its use should be carefully considered and circumscribed. Generally, I only suggest its use during the premenstruum when Heat, Dampness, and Stagnation are at their height. After menstruation, *Fu Zheng* or supporting the Righteous therapies should be used in order to promote the generation of New Flesh.

1) Si Yao You Gao (Four Medicinal Oil Paste)

The escarotic suppository I currently use is called Si Yao Yo Gao (Four Medicinal Oil Paste). It is a combination of Chinese and Western medicinals. Its ingredients are:

> Radix Angelicae Sinensis
> Pulvis Indigo
> Radix Symphyti Officinalis
> Fructus Bruceae Javanicae
> Acacia Catechu
> Cod Liver Oil
> Oleum Melaleucae Linariifoliae
> Oleum Thujae Occidentalis
> Oleum Sesami
> Lard
> Beeswax

Sesame Oil, Lard, and Beeswax are the vehicle or medium for

this suppository. However, all three are considered nourishing to Yin substance. Dang Gui, Indigo, and Brucea are all standard Chinese ingredients and have already been described above. Acacia Catechu is originally an East Indian medicinal. Its TCM description is that it drains Dampness, absorbs seepage, stops bleeding, stops *Dai Xia*, and generates New Flesh. The other four ingredients are Western medicinals and, therefore, merit individual attention.

Oleum Melaleucae Linariifoliae is Tea Tree Oil. It is the Australian version of Cajeput Oil with which it is almost identical. It is Acrid, Bitter, and Hot and enters the Lung, Large Intestine, and Spleen Channels. Tea Tree Oil clears Heat and dissolves Toxins, kills Worms, activates the Blood, disperses Stagnations and Accumulations, and stops pain. It is primarily used externally. It is a specific against papilloma virus.

Oleum Thujae Occidentalis is Thuja Oil. It is Bitter, Acrid, Astringent, and slightly Cold. It cools the Blood, stops bleeding, promotes the generation of New Flesh, and is used topically for its specific anti-papilloma effect.

If one reads the label on a bottle of Vitamin A soft gelatin capsules, one will see that the liquid inside is none other than Cod Liver Oil. Therefore, in this formula, Cod Liver Oil is used as an inexpensive and readily available source of Vitamin A. Vitamin A tonifies the Blood and benefits the *Jing* Essence. It brightens the eyes and nourishes the skin. It clears Heat from the Blood and treats Deficiency Fire Patterns. As such, it is a *Qing Xue* ingredient similar to those listed above.

Radix Symphyti Officinalis (Comfrey Root) is Bitter, Sweet, Astringent, and Cool. It enters the Liver, Lungs, Stomach, and Large Intestine Channels. It cools the Blood, clears Heat from the Liver, transforms Phlegm and stops cough (especially Dry

Phlegm Cough), promotes the circulation of Blood and disperses Stagnant Blood, promotes the generation of New Flesh, soothes the *Jin* Sinews, knits and strengthens the bones, clears and eliminates Damp Heat in the Lower Burner, and astringes the Two Yin (i.e. the anus and urethra).

This formula's TCM functions as a whole are to clear Heat, dissolve Toxins, kill Worms (i.e. parasites, not necessarily worms *per se*), activate and nourish the Blood, disperse Stagnation and Accumulation, and generate New Flesh. In addition, Pulvis Indigo is specifically anti-viral and Brucea, Thuja Oil, and Tea Tree Oil have all demonstrated anti-wart virus activity. Based on TCM therapeutic methodology, Dang Gui, Sesame Oil, Lard, and Comfrey are all *Fu Zheng* ingredients included to mollify the otherwise potentially harsh effects of the *Qu Xie* ingredients.

This suppository can be applied to the cervix either with an intravaginal applicator or on the head of a tampon at night before bed. If it is applied and held in place with a tampon, the tampon should be removed in the morning upon arising. According to my protocols, this escarotic suppository is used nightly for from 1-3 months from midcycle to the onset of menstruation. Appendix III contains the naturopathic guidelines for escarotic therapy based on the staging of cervical disease. It should be noted, however, that this naturopathic approach to escarosis is more caustic than my protocol and, therefore, is repeated less often. In addition, the Vag Packs (short for Vaginal Depletion Packs) described in this appendix are inserted by the ND during an office visit, whereas my patients are able to insert the suppositories themselves at home.

2) Acidophilus Suppositories

For clearing and eliminating more obvious Damp Heat, I

typically use either of two very similar suppositories both made with Lactobacillus Acidophilus. The first method is to mix 3 drops of Metagenics' Mycelized Children's Multiple Vitamins into one packet of Metagenics' Ultradophilus. This is stirred into a paste, placed on the head of a slender tampon, and inserted into the vagina BID. The second method is to mix one packet of Ultradophilus into a teaspoon of room temperature, non-fat milk. Stir into a paste and allow to sit for 1/2 hour. Apply to the head of a tampon and insert BID.

The above two clearing and eliminating Damp Heat suppositories are used mostly during the premenstruum when Dampness and Heat tend to accumulate below or at any time when *Dai Xia* becomes an issue. These two methods are specifically for *Bai Dai* or White *Dai* which is curdy like cottage cheese. Usually with this type of discharge there will be little or no vaginal inflammation or irritation. This type of *Dai* is due to a combination of Damp Heat and *Chong* or parasites. This is supported by Han Bai-ling, a famous, now retired, TCM gynecologist in Haerbin. Dr. Han, in *Bai Ling Fu Ke*, gives a prescription for the treatment of *Dai Xia* which is a suppository made from a piece of raw meat in which are wrapped *Jie Du* ingredients. Dr. Han says that the *Chong* will enter the raw meat and be killed by the poisons within, thus eliminating the *Dai Xia*.[13] Worms *per se* do not cause *Dai Xia; Jun* or yeast and microbes do. This, I think, substantiates my hypothesis that yeast should be subsumed under the *Chong* category of *Bu Nei Bu Wai Yin* and, therefore, should be treated by specifically *Sha Jun* or killing yeast anti-microbial therapy.

3) Borax Suppositories

If the *Dai* is more obviously yellow accompanied by irritation and inflammation, another suppository which is very effective is to fill Double "O" gelatin capsules with powdered Boric Acid available at most drug stores. These are inserted one at a time.

The gelatin will dissolve and the Boric Acid (i.e. Borax) will clear Heat, eliminate Dampness, and dissolve Toxins. This method usually makes short work of *Huang Dai* of recent or recurrent onset.

4) *Fu Zheng* Suppositories

The three *Fu Zheng* suppositories which I use to promote the growth of New Tissue are Cod Liver Oil on the head of a tampon, Liquid Folate on the head of a tampon, and egg whites applied to sterile cotton and inserted with a tampon or intravaginal applicator. All three promote the growth of healthy New Tissue. They are used after the period when Blood is being replenished and after any courses of escarotic therapy but before having a new Pap. The TCM description of Folic Acid is given below under orthomolecular therapy. The TCM description of Vitamin A has been given above.

C) Vaginal Douches

Vaginal douches are yet another topical treatment which can be used adjunctively in the treatment of CIN and related pathologies. I use douches for two main purposes: 1) to promote the growth of healthy New Tissue and to mitigate the effects of harsh *Qu Xie* therapy, and 2) to clear and eliminate Damp Heat manifesting as *Dai Xia*.

1) Comfrey Root Douche

This douche is for the generation of New Flesh and to mitigate any damage to healthy tissue done by *Qu Xie* or escarotic therapies. A strong decoction of Comfrey Root is made and allowed to cool to body temperature. This is put into a douche bag or vaginal syringe and is used to irrigate the vagina and cervix. I prescribe Comfrey Root douches in the mornings after removal of escarotic suppositories or when any *Qu Xie* therapy has caused irritation and inflammation. The TCM functions of Comfrey Root are to cool the Blood, stop bleeding, clear Heat from the Liver, transform Phlegm, stop cough, promote the circulation of Blood, disperse Stagnant Blood, generate New Tissue, soothe the *Jin* Sinews, knit and strengthen the bones, clear and eliminate Damp Heat from the Lower Burner, and astringe the Two *Yin*.

2) Dai Xia Douche

Dai Xia Douche is for the adjunctive treatment of *Dai Xia* due to flourishing of Damp Hot Toxins. Its ingredients are:

>Fructus Cnidii Monnieri
>Acacia Catechu
>Alumen
>Borax
>Myrrha

These ingredients are decocted in water and the decoction is allowed to cool to body temperature. The liquid is strained and put in a douche bag or vaginal syringe. It is used to irrigate the vagina. This is an extremely effective formula for the treatment of Damp Heat *Dai* and is recommended whenever such Abnormal Vaginal Discharge accompanies a

patient's cervical dysplasia. It can be used for either *Bai Dai* or *Huang Dai*.

D) Abdominal Compresses & Plasters

When Stagnant Blood is a prominent complicating factor in an individual woman's TCM *Zheng* with or without cervical dysplasia, I frequently employ abdominal compresses and plasters adjunctively. The two main treatments I use are Tiao Jing Gao and Castor Oil Compresses.

1) Tiao Jing Gao (Period Regulating Plaster)

Tiao Jing Gao is comprised of powdered herbs mixed with vinegar and stirred into a paste. This paste is made into thin discs approximately the size of a quarter. These are applied to Shen Que (CV 8) and Extra points Zi Gong Xue (1 *Cun* lateral to Gui Lai (St 29)). A square adhesive bandage is used to keep these in place for 24 hours. These plasters are replaced daily. Depending upon the patient's constitution and tone of the striae (*Cou Li*) of their skin, these plasters may cause skin irritation which is not wholly unwanted. If such irritation occurs, it may be treated according to the protocols given in *A Handbook of Traditional Chinese Dermatology* for *Gao Yao Feng* or Plant & Contact Dermatitis.[14]

When patients have pronounced *Tong Jing* or Painful Menstruation or other complicating signs and symptoms of Stagnant Blood, Tiao Jing Gao can be used during the premenstruum and even during the first 24 hours of the flow itself. This *Gao* helps to continue treatment throughout the day and night during the time when Qi and Blood become most Stagnant, mobilizing these for discharge during the period itself. This technique is especially useful if the patient cannot receive intensive acupuncture during the premenstruum.

The ingredients in Tiao Jing Gao are:

    Gummum Olibani
    Myrrha
    Pulvis Radicis Paeoniae Albae
    Pulvis Radicis Achyranthis
    Pulvis Radicis Salviae Miltorrhizae
    Pulvis Fructi Crataegi

Pulvis Radicis Saussureae Seu Vladimiriae
Pulvis Floris Carthami
Borneolum

2) Castor Oil Compresses

Castor Oil (Oleum Semenis Ricinis Communis) activates the Blood, disperses Stagnation and Accumulation, promotes bowel movements, and raises prolapse. Castor Oil compresses are another useful adjunctive therapy for Stagnant Qi and Blood. They can be used for any hypochondral or abdominal masses (*Zheng Jia Ji Ju*) due to Stagnant Qi and Blood. They are done at home by the patient and can be used to extend the effects of intensive premenstrual acupuncture or in place of this depending upon the patient's needs. In addition to being a therapeutically effective therapy, Castor Oil compresses are a good way to enlist and encourage the patient's involvement in their treatment.

Castor Oil is warmed in a pan. At the same time, several slices of fresh Ginger are simmered in 1 1/2 quarts of water for 7-10 minutes. A thick layer of Castor Oil is applied to the abdomen from the umbilicus to the pubic hair. This is then covered by a towel dipped in the Ginger tea and wrung out. This towel should be applied as hot as possible without undue discomfort to the patient. This can be covered by a hot water bottle and a blanket to ensure continuous warmth and protection from chill. This compress should be left in place from 15-20 minutes and can be repeated daily or every other day during the premenstruum.

E) Herbal Enemas

Medicated enemas made from freshly decocted, ground roasted coffee are a final useful adjunctive therapy in some cases of CIN. These are used to clear Heat and Stagnation from the Liver and Large Intestine. These two Organs have a close reciprocal relationship via the Five Phase *Ke* cycle. Coffee enemas are another way the patient can extend the range of their therapy at home. They are especially useful if there is Liver Qi complicated by bowel problems, such as flatulence, diarrhea, and constipation. Their use should be co-ordinated with the premenstruum so as to achieve maximum dispersion and discharge without injuring the *Zheng Qi*. This is the only way coffee should be used by human beings.

ORTHOMOLECULAR THERAPY

Orthomolecular is a term coined by Dr. Linus Pauling. The Greek prefix *ortho* has almost exactly the same meaning in this case as the Chinese term *Zheng*: righteous, normal, or regular. Orthomolecular therapy means the therapeutic supplementation of the same molecules which constitute the body. It is the technical name for what most people commonly think of as vitamin therapy. However, orthomolecular therapy consists of more than just supplementing vitamins and minerals. It also consists of supplementing amino acids, enzymes, co-enzymes, co-factors, and essential fatty acids.

Here in the United States, most practitioners of TCM consider orthomolecular therapy outside their scope of practice. However, use of vitamins at least has been a part of Chinese acupuncture for the last 20 years in *Shui Zhen* or Water Needle therapy. There is no reason why vitamins, minerals, amino acids, fatty acids, and enzymes cannot be described according to the rubric and administered according to the methodology of TCM.

Personally, it is my opinion that American patients are subject to so much emotional, dietary, and environmental stress that

Chinese herbal medicine alone is often not completely satisfactory for the treatment of our modern, complex *Zheng* caused by *Bing Yin* unknown when most Chinese medicine was developed. Orthomolecular supplements are powerful and effective with a relatively high benefit/risk ratio. Since Chinese herbal medicinals themselves are nothing other than vitamins, minerals, amino acids, enzymes, fatty acids, proteins, carbohydrates, and sugars, I see no good conceptual reason for modern orthomolecular therapy not to be included in rational TCM practice.

There does exist a standard orthomolecular therapy for cervical dysplasia which has been used with great success by American naturopaths. It is given in Pizzorno & Murray's *A Textbook of Natural Medicine, Vol. I*, a standard naturopathic clinical manual.[15] Pizzorno & Murray's orthomolecular protocol consists of:

Folic Acid	10 mg p.d. for 3 mos.
B_6	50 mg TID
B_{12}	1 mg QID
Beta-carotene	200,000 IU p.d.
Vitamin C	1 g + p.d.
Vitamin E	200IU QID
Selenium	400 mcg p.d.
Zinc Picolinate	30 mg p.d.

These doses can be obtained at a cost of approximately $2.00 per day by taking the following products manufactured and distributed by Metagenics:

Chlorotene	1 tablet TID
Intrinsi B_{12}/Folate	1 tablet BID
Multigenics	2 tablets TID
Zinc Picolinate	1 tablet BID

Plus 1 drop per day of Papillon (30ml Folate) available from Scientific Botanicals in Seattle, WA.

The TCM functions of each of the ingredients in this protocol are:

Folic Acid nourishes the Blood, relaxes the Liver, calms the *Hun*, and secures the fetus. It enters the Liver Channel.

B$_6$ enters the Liver/Gallbladder. It clears Heat, extinguishes Wind, harmonizes Wood and Earth, relieves depression, clears Heat from the Stomach and Damp Heat from the Liver/Gallbladder.

B$_{12}$ tonifies the Qi to transform the Blood and benefits the Spleen.

Beta-carotene clears Heat, cools the Blood, invigorates the Blood and dispels Stagnation, activates the Qi and stops pain, expels Wind and moves the Blood in Wind Damp *Bi*, transforms Phlegm in Lung Heat cough and asthma in children and adults, combats cancer, and disperses Nodulation.

Vitamin C clears Heat and dissolves Toxins, clears Heat from the Heart and calms the *Shen*.

Vitamin E tonifies Yang, nourishes Liver Blood, tonifies Kidney Yang, benefits the *Jing* Essence, and nourishes the *Jin* Sinews.

Selenium benefits Yin, restrains Floating Yang, settles and calms the Spirit, and astringes the Essence. It enters the Liver and Kidney Channels.

Zinc benefits the *Jing* Essence, nourishes the Blood, strengthens the bones, brightens the eyes, and specifically tonifies the

Jing so as to support the Righteous in order to hold Evil in check.

Based on the above TCM descriptions of the individual medicinals in this protocol, we can then describe the overall therapeutic effects of this protocol just as if it were any other TCM herbal formula. As a TCM formula, this combination of vitamins and minerals nourishes the Blood and cools it, activates the Qi and dredges the Liver, nourishes the Blood to relax Liver, harmonizes Wood and Earth, benefits the *Jing* Essence, clears Heat, eliminates Dampness, and dissolves Toxins. Therefore, its TCM rationale is somewhat similar to both Dan Zhi Xiao Yao San and Health Concern's Astra Isatis.

I have found the combination of Chinese herbal medicine and orthomolecular supplements well received by my patients with a high degree of compliance. I have had only a single patient who did not get a negative Pap within 3 months of starting such a combined regime of Chinese herbal and orthomolecular therapies. This woman began with a diagnosis of areas of both severe and moderate dysplasia. After 3 months, this woman's severe dysplasia was downgraded to moderate and the moderate dysplasia had disappeared.

If the patient also suffers from periodic outbreaks of HSV II or herpes genitalia, I often add to this regime Organic Germanium (Ge-132), 50 mg BID. This is to further nourish the Blood and *Jing* and tonify the Kidneys so as to hold the virus in check or latency. As a TCM medicinal, Organic Germanium nourishes Liver Blood and tonifies Kidney Yang. Therefore, it strengthens the Kidney *Jing*. This medicinal is a Yang tonic and is Warm. It should be used only with care and at low doses in patients with Excess Heat unless combined with other Heat-clearing medicinals. When used by young, relatively robust patients, Organic Germanium should only be added to the regime when one is run down or fatigued or when there are prodromal signs and symptoms of an incipient outbreak. It is available from Bioenergy Nutrients of Boulder, CO.

ACUPUNCTURE

When women come to me with cervical dysplasia, I typically administer acupuncture intensively during the week before each period for the first 3 periods. As mentioned above, this is when any Dampness, Heat, or Stagnant Qi and Blood are at their maximum concentration in the Lower Burner. The period itself is a discharge of Excess. Therefore, working in consonance with the body's periodicity, this is the most effective time to promote discharge of Evil Qi. This is also the most effective time to treat any menopathies due to Evil Excesses. By intensive acupuncture, I mean treating every other day for 3-4 treatments, the last treatment being administered on day 1 of the new cycle if there is dysmenorrhea or on the last day of the old cycle if there is not.

Most menopathies can be treated in 3 menstrual cycles using a combination of dietary therapy, exercise, deep relaxation, herbs, orthomoleculars, and acupuncture. The menstruation is a monthly report card on the female patient's state of health and is especially indicative of the pelvic environment. Above I said that the first thing to address in the TCM treatment of dysplasia are any menstrual abnormalities or *Dai Xia*. Once such *Yue Jing Bing* and *Dai Xia* have been treated successfully, the majority of women will also get a good or clean Pap. Therefore, it is during this initial 3 month period that I make maximum use of acupuncture. This, in turn, enables the patient to make maximum efficient use of her time and money.

Because the TCM treatment of cervical dysplasia is first aimed at rebalancing the patient's TCM disease categories and *Zheng*, an acupuncture protocol should be formulated on that basis.

In other words, I choose points to treat *Tong Jing* or Painful Menstruation due to Stagnant Qi and Blood or Depressive Liver Heat if that is the patient's TCM diagnosis. I have no special miracle points for the treatment of cervical dysplasia *per se*. If there is premenstrual *Dai Xia*, I treat for that. If there is premenstrual *Shao Fu Tong* or Lower Abdominal Pain, I treat for that. If there is PMS, I treat for that picking points on the basis of the patient's *Zheng* and her presenting signs and symptoms. This is the basic approach of TCM acupuncture. A further description of this point selection methodology is given in my *Sticking to the Point, a Rational Methodology for the Step By Step Formulation & Administration of an Acupuncture Treatment*.[16]

When creating such a TCM acupuncture protocol, typically several *Zhu Xue* or Commanding points are selected based on the *Zheng* to be rectified. To these are added several *Bei Xue* or subsidiary points. These are local points of symptomatic action or distant points of specific, empirical action. Below is a list of Extra points useful in the treatment of gynecological problems often encountered in women presenting with cervical dysplasia. These points are taken from two famous Taiwanese practitioners, Tung Ching-chang[17] and Li Su-huai.[18] These points are not discussed in the more popular acupuncture point books and I have found them quite useful in my clinical practice.

NON-MERIDIAN ACUPOINTS USEFUL IN THE TREATMENT OF CIN

Wooden Woman (Mu Fu)

Location: 0.3 *Cun* lateral from the center of the dorsum of the distal phalangeal joint of the second toe

Indications: Leukorrhea, dysmenorrhea, amenorrhea, infertility, & PID due to Liver Qi Stagnation

Method: Perpendicular insertion, 0.2-0.4 *Cun* in depth

Return to Nest (Huan Chao)

Location: 0.5 *Cun* to the ulnar side from the center of the ventral surface of the middle phalanx of the ring finger

Indications: Leukorrhea, uterine tumor, frequent miscarriage, retroversion of the uterus

Method: Needle the right side only in a woman, 0.3 *Cun* deep perpendicularly

Gynecological Points (Fu Ke Xue)

Location: On the ulnar side of the dorsal proximal phalanx of the thumb. 2 points on each thumb for a total of 4 points bilaterally. If the phalanx is divided into thirds, the points are located 0.3 and 0.6 *Cun* distal to the metacarpal-phalangeal joint.

Indications: Endometrioma, infertility, irregular menstruation, menorrhagia, dysmenorrhea, and uterine pain due to Stagnant Blood

Method: Perpendicular insertion, 0.25 *Cun* in depth

White Cloud (Yun Bai)

Location: 2.5 *Cun* below the acromion process and 1.5 *Cun* anterior

Indications: Vaginal inflammation, vaginal itching, vaginal pain, leukorrhea

Method: Perpendicular insertion, 0.3-0.5 *Cun* in depth

Cancer Root Two (Ai Gen Er)

Location: From the junction of the cuneiform and 1st metatarsal, draw a line laterally across the bottom of the foot at a right angle to the midline of the sole. This point is located on this line 1 finger-breadth from the medial edge of the sole.

Indications: Cancer of the esophagus, rectum, cervix, or lymphnodes

Method: Perpendicular insertion 0.3-0.5 *Cun* in depth. Numbness and soreness should be generated to the toe.

After the first 3 months of intensive acupuncture during the premenstruum, most of my dysplasia patients have minimal menstrually-related signs and symptoms. What signs and symptoms are usually left are minimal enough not to require acupuncture treatment. If the patient wants to continue acupuncture therapy because they appreciate its benefits, I switch to more *Ben* or Root treatments administered only once every several weeks. Since I treat with a full panoply of healing modalities, I do not feel compelled to treat all my patients all the time with acupuncture. After the initial 3 months, most patients are doing well enough that their Three Free Therapies, herbal medicine, and orthomolecular therapy are all they need. In a few cases, where CIN is more severe, including carcinoma in situ, intensive acupuncture may be necessary for more than just the first 3 cycles. However, this is the exception rather than the rule.

I have only been able to find a single clinical report on the efficacy of acupuncture in treating the uterine cervix in the English language acupuncture literature. This is in *Advances in Acupuncture and Anesthesia* published in Beijing in 1980. In an article entitled "Acupuncture Treatment of Cervical Erosion" by Liang Rui-jun *et al.*, 1010 women with cervical erosion were needled at Xia Yi Xue.[19] This specifically refers to needling transcutaneously upwards from San Yin Jiao (Sp 6) 1-1.5 *Cun*. Cervical erosion, if that indeed was these women's actual Western medical diagnosis, is not cervical dysplasia. (Unless this diagnosis was mistranslated into English.) However, this report does at least suggest that acupuncture can be an effective treatment for cervical problems.

Of these 1010 women, 419 suffered from 1st degree erosion, 467 from 2nd degree erosion, and 124 from 3rd degree erosion. 630 were subsequently cured, 280 improved, and 100 failed to respond to this treatment. There was 92% overall effectiveness for women with 1st and 2nd degree erosion, and 75% overall effectiveness for women with 3rd degree erosion. In considering these results, it should be kept in mind that only one point was needled bilaterally and that not on the basis of individual *Bian Zheng* but, presumably, on the basis of *Bian Bing*. Also, Sp 6 was not needled perpendicularly as it usually is. It is my opinion that a more numerous selection and employment of points based on individualized *Bian Zheng* diagnosis and needled more standardly would achieve even better success rates. Nevertheless, even the rates achieved in this clinical trial seem quite good.

VISUALIZATION & INCANTATION

Ever since the authors of the Ma Wang Tui manuscripts at the latest (circa 200 BCE) and continuing up through the Qing

Dynasty and the Republic on the mainland and still today in overseas Chinese communities, many Chinese doctors have concomitantly recommended shamanic methods of healing in tandem with herbs, diet, and acupuncture. The term *Xie Qi* or Evil Qi harkens back to the shamanic stage in the development of Chinese medicine, a stage that has never been eradicated in the minds of the Chinese folk. *Xie* means evil but also means evil spirit or demon in Chinese. In shamanic medicine, disease is due to attack by evil spirits. In Asia, it is widely believed that pestilential diseases are due to spirit attack and that pestilential diseases effecting the skin in particular are due to a class of spirits called *Naga* in Sanskrit, *Lu* in Tibetan, and *Long* in Chinese. These are serpent or dragon spirits which live under the ground and in lakes, rivers, and bodies of water and who jealously guard there hidden treasures.

Buddhism has developed a number of methods for controlling the predation of such Nagas. Acting on a large societal scale, the erection of *Ta* or pagodas is one way Chinese have sought to control evil Nagas. Individually, there are a number of *sadhana* or ritual *cum* mantra *cum* meditation practices which seek to confer power over marauding Nagas. In particular, in Tantric Buddhism, the sadhanas of Vajrapani, Garuda, and the Three Wrathful Lords (Drak Sum Gonpo) are especially designed to negate the evil, disease-carrying influences of these serpent spirits.

Personally, I have found these sadhanas to be very helpful in treating viral diseases. They can be done by both the physician and the patient. Such sadhanas were traditionally considered essential parts of the education and development of Buddhist medical practitioners in Central and Northern Asia. They are not something that can be transmitted or learned from a book such as this, but they can be learned from certain Tibetan Lamas living and actively teaching in the United States.

In lieu of such traditional Buddhist shamanic methods of visualization and incantation, patients can also employ more contemporary Western methods of visualization to good purpose in the treatment of CIN. For further specifics concerning healing visualization technique, readers are referred to O.Carl Simonton *et al.*'s *Getting Well Again*.[20] Written by a husband/wife team of cancer therapists, this book outlines a step by step program of therapeutic visualization which can be modified to treat any disease and which can accommodate the beliefs of almost any patient. Visualization is an important approach to healing of which all patients and practitioners should be aware.

In our clinic, we employ an NLP practitioner to help deal with this aspect of our patients' healing. NLP stands for Neurolinguistic Programming. It is a system of psychotherapy designed to modify behavior by modifying our beliefs. Instead of analyzing one's feelings about an issue, the NLP practitioner identifies the subconscious beliefs about one's problems and then seeks to supplant these unworkable beliefs with ones which are more pragmatic, healthy, and positive. First, the NLP practitioner ascertains the patient's dominant mode of relating to reality, whether visual, auditory, tactile, etc. Then, through other techniques derived in part from hypnotherapy and visualization, he or she helps the patient create a new *mythos* for that aspect of their life for which they are seeking help.

One of the techniques NLP practitioners use has to do with catalyzing what Hippocrates called the *Vis Mediatrix Naturae* or the healing power of nature. When we cut ourselves or catch a cold, we automatically assume that these are temporary problems which will without doubt heal. We may be temporarily uncomfortable but we tend not to worry or doubt whether or not we will get better. Without much thought or even any thought, the wound closes and disappears or the cold goes away without any long-term sequelae. However, when we receive a diagnosis of a chronic or life-threatening disease, our minds are filled with doubt, negativity, and pessimism. We may have been told by a health care professional or another authority our condition is intractable, incurable, or recalcitrant. Or, seeing others with the same condition, we assume that our disease will run the same depressing and frustrating course.

However, how we view our diseases, how we imagine them, frame them, feel them, and conceive of them has a very profound effect on how we ultimately experience them and their course. Through NLP, our stories or myths about our disease can be reframed, repatterned, and retold in such a way as to catalyze the same spontaneous healing energy we assume when we cut our finger or sprain our ankle. In our clinic, we have found such NLP reframing to be of utmost importance when dealing with diseases such as HIV, HSV, HPV, cancer, MS, SLE, and other such diseases which, in most peoples' minds, are conceived to be intractable, incurable, and hopeless. By changing one's conception of their disease, their personal script or storyline is rewritten and, in the process, the *Vis Mediatrix Naturae* is catalyzed.

SEX DURING REMEDIAL TREATMENT

Sex is a healthy discharge of Yang Qi. Orgasm can release pent-up Liver Qi and can be therapeutic. However, sex can also cause problems if not understood and approached carefully.

First of all, there should be no deep vaginal penetration during any escarotic therapy. This can cause further trauma and inflammation of the cervix. Secondly, there should be no genital sex during menstruation. This causes retroversion up and in of the downward discharging Blood resulting in Stagnant

Qi and Blood. Although many women with Liver Qi may experience an increase of sexual desire during their period due to an increase of Liver Heat and, therefore, *Ming Men* Fire, it is not healthy to act upon this desire in that way. Third, all vaginal penetration should be accompanied by the use of condoms. It should be assumed that one's sexual partner *is* infected with HPV and monilia. Unprotected sex only allows for further repeated infection. This is especially important since most men infected with HPV and monilia or genital tract candidiasis are asymptomatic. According to Dr. Larry Lipshultz:

> The incidence of subclinical HPV infection (i.e. invisible infection) in male consorts of women with condyloma is high. In one group of 57 men, 95% were found to have condyloma. 90% had subclinical (invisible) disease.[21]

Until women with cervical dysplasia achieve a negative Pap smear, their partners should always be required to use condoms during genital sex. Until that time, it should be assumed that their immune system is incompetent and that reinfection may occur. After a negative Pap smear has been obtained, women in monogamous relationships may engage in unprotected sex based on the assumption that their immune system is now competent to deal with HPV. However, if the woman takes a new lover, extreme caution is advised since she may be exposing herself to a new strain of HPV for which she does not carry antibodies.

Moderate, protected sex at times other than during escarotic therapy and the period is permissible. However, the emphasis should be on clitoral stimulation as opposed to deep, forceful vaginal penetration. In general, women are not as easily depleted by orgasm as are men since they do not lose their *Jing* in the same way. Nevertheless, women do consume Yin during sex and do discharge and dissipate their Qi. This is what is so liberating and relaxing about orgasm. Therefore, since maintenance of sufficient Kidney *Jing* is an issue in any disease complicated by a Warm Hidden Evil, CIN patients are advised on sexual moderation.

TREATMENT OF SEXUAL PARTNERS

The above caution regarding repeated reinfection by one's sexual partner brings up the issue of whether one's partner should be treated. It is logical to assume that reinfection will occur if sex is not protected and few persons relish the habitual use of condoms. Therefore, it is also logical that one's partner should, indeed, be treated simultaneously. Although this is logical and most of my patients query me about or even suggest this approach, the problem is that it is difficult to diagnose asymptomatic HPV infection in men without the presence of visible genital warts.

Recently, my office staff surveyed the urologists in our area as to whether they did HPV DNA probe testing and whether they treated men with asymptomatic infections which could not be diagnosed colposcopically. All the urologists queried responded that they did not do HPV DNA testing nor did they offer any treatment for those men infected asymptomatically. Several of the office staff of these urologists mentioned that our query is a frequently asked one. One area gynecologist mentioned that dermatologists may be more interested in and open to attempting to treat asymptomatic HPV infection. HPV DNA testing is done by a lab in Denver, but even the STD clinic at Denver General Hospital, the largest in the Denver metro area, does not offer treatment for anything other than colposcopically visible lesions.

I, on the other hand, do recommend that my female patients'

sexual partners come in so that we can inspect them for visible genital warts and test them Vega biokinesiologically (VBK) for the presence of HPV. Inspection of the genitalia for warts may reveal obvious, large condylomatous growths. However, often it does not. The next step is to apply vinegar to the penis and inspect it with magnification under light. Warty tissue will be revealed as brighter, white areas by this technique called aceto-white staining. However, even this method often reveals nothing. One further technique is to do Vega biokinesiological testing using homeopathic nosodes of HPV as resonance filters (VBK). This is a type of muscle testing which can reveal the presence of viruses difficult to detect by other means. This method, although not as conclusive to some as taking a swab from the urethra and doing a DNA probe test, is easy to do without pain or embarrassment and I feel is accurate when performed correctly.

If a man has gross or visible genital warts, these should be removed by a Western MD if possible. If such cell-destructive or surgical removal is ineffective, immune-modulating therapy, whether Western or Chinese, can be used to increase success rates. See the following section on the treatment of genital warts for further information on this. If the presence of HPV is revealed solely by VBK testing with the use of resonance filters, treatment of the partner should proceed based upon the regimes given in the following section of this book on the preventive treatment of prostrate problems. Primarily, such treatment consists of composite homotoxicological, orthomolecular, and herbal remedies, such as Power Mushrooms and Bioradiance, until the man tests negative for HPV.

DURATION OF REMEDIAL TREATMENT

In general, the duration of remedial therapy for CIN utilizing the comprehensive treatment plan outlined above lasts as long as it takes to treat any TCM disease associated with the period or with Abnormal Vaginal Discharge. This can include the following list of Chinese *Yue Jing Bing* or menopathies:

Yue Jing Xian Qi	Menstruation Ahead of Schedule
Yue Jing Hou Qi	Menstruation After Schedule
Yu Jing Bu Tiao	Irregular Menstruation
Yue Jing Guo Duo	Excessive Menstrual Flow
Yue Jing Guo Shao	Scanty Menstrual Flow
Tong Jing	Painful Menstruation
Jing Xing Ru Fang Zhang Tong	Premenstrual Breast Distention (&) Pain
Dai Xia	Abnormal Vaginal Discharge
Beng Lou	Abnormal or Dysfunctional Uterine Bleeding

In my experience, these are the main categories of Chinese gynecological diseases associated with cervical dysplasia. Most of these can be treated most of the time in from 3-4 menstrual cycles *if*:

1) the *Bian Zheng* diagnosis is correct

2) the treatment is correct

3) the patient complies with the treatment as scheduled

These are three big ifs. Nevertheless, if the gynecopathies

above are rectified, this means without doubt that the internal environment of the pelvis has been brought to a state of relative health. As mentioned above, there is humoral or hormonal regulation of the immune system. Regulation of the menstrual cycle and rebalancing of any menopathies obviously means that a woman's hormones have been brought into balance as well. This, in turn, suggests that that woman's humoral immune response has also returned to a healthy state and is now able to maintain any remaining HPV in a latent state. This is a very important point which should not be overlooked by TCM practitioners who may not be aware of this relationship between a woman's periods, her hormones, and her humoral immune response. At this point, it is safe to recommend a repeat Pap smear in order to confirm whether or not the dysplasia has gone into remission.

SCHEDULING REPEAT PAP SMEARS

Scheduling repeat Pap smears is an important issue. They should be done in the week after the period, not during the week before. There is a better chance of getting a good or negative Pap after any Stagnation and Accumulation has been discharged. There is more probability of a good Pap at this time than when Liver Qi and Stagnant Blood are at their height and consequently Dampness and Heat. However, this statement implies that one good Pap smear does not constitute a lifetime cure. The patient must be counselled to continue a preventive maintenance regime to prevent relapse or recurrence. It is my opinion that, since we are dealing with a Warm Hidden Evil disease, a negative Pap may constitute only a remission. On the other hand, with proper preventive care, this remission can continue indefinitely or at least well into old age.

CHAPTER FOUR
COMPLICATIONS ENCOUNTERED DURING REMEDIAL TREATMENT OF CIN

There are three important complications in the remedial treatment of CIN beyond failure of patient compliance to the Three Free Therapies and patients going out of town during their premenstruum. These three complicating factors are polysystemic chronic candidiasis (PSCC), amoebiasis, and herpes genitalia (HSV II). Each of these require, I believe, specific discussion and treatment.

CANDIDIASIS

Due to our poor modern American diet, widespread use of antibiotics, environmental pollution, stress, and the use of oral contraceptives and steroids, many Americans and especially women are being overgrown by the yeast Candida Albicans. This commensal fungus is a saprophyte which is present in all human beings. Its proliferation is normally kept in check by the body's immune system. However, the various disease factors listed above can all contribute to a runaway proliferation of this yeast which can then release large quantities of toxins into the system. It can also upset the hormonal balance and depress the immune system, thus allowing other pathogens, such as bacteria, protozoa, and viruses, to proliferate and also cause disease.

Because men in general visit doctors less often and, therefore, take less antibiotics, and because they do not use OCs, men have a lesser incidence of PSCC. In addition, women's hormonal fluctuations cyclically and during pregnancy also allow for easier candida overgrowth due to the close relationship of the immune system to hormonal control. In women, PSCC can contribute to a wide variety of signs and symptoms, such as *Dai Xia*, PMS, dysmenorrhea, infertility, depression, frigidity, migraines, diarrhea, flatulence, constipation, cystitis, and vaginal and anal pruritus. Not only do hormonal fluctuations allow for yeast overgrowth, but yeast themselves secrete toxins which further imbalance the hormonal system thus enabling them to foil the body's immune system. Therefore, many female problems according to Western medicine associated with hormonal imbalance can, in part, be due to candidiasis.

It is not uncommon to find women with cervical dysplasia who also suffer from chronic candidiasis. Such women typically have weak Spleen function according to TCM and Damp Heat in their Lower Burners. Chinese medicine believes that *Chong* or parasites arise from Damp Heat or at least that Damp Heat provides a conducive internal environment for their arisal. Although Chinese herbal medicine treats both Spleen Deficiency and Damp Heat, patients whose cases are complicated by parasites, including candida, tend not to respond as expected to simply tonifying the Spleen, clearing Heat, and eliminating Dampness. Although their TCM *Bian Zheng* diagnosis seems clear-cut if complicated, they often do not show marked improvement with the standard TCM treatment for these Patterns. However, if candidiasis is indicated by the constellation of their signs and symptoms and they are treated additionally and specifically to *Sha Jun* or kill yeast,[1] they often do make remarkable progress. This is an important point which must be stressed in modern clinical practice.

These women tend to have numerous and ever-shifting signs

and symptoms. Although their TCM Patterns are capable of being parsed out and described, yet the severity and multiplicity of their signs and symptoms seem disproportionate. They respond only very slowly and incompletely to traditional Chinese herbal therapy, and because their digestion is chronically out of balance, much time and energy is spent trying to deal with that before being able to address their menopathies and the CIN itself. Since all internally administered herbal medicine must go through the digestion, chronically imbalanced digestion is a stumbling block to further herbal therapy.

When I come across such patients who have chronic loose stools, recurrent yeasty discharges before their periods, more severe PMS, fatigue, depression, anxiety, and irritability, who binge on sweats and crave carbohydrates, and whose right *Chi* or Foot position pulse is deeper superficially than their left though wiry and even slippery deeper down, I tend to suspect candidiasis. In terms of the Four (Methods of) diagnosis, questioning can help confirm this diagnosis. If such patients have a history of antibiotic, steroid, or oral contraceptive use, these *Bing Yin* also suggest an increased likelihood of candidiasis. There are non-traditional diagnostic methods to also confirm this diagnosis, such as biokinesiology with potentized resonance filters and dark field, live cell microscopy. I have been experimenting with the first of these and attempting to corroborate my kinesiological findings with my pulse readings and, although it is still too early to say conclusively, I feel I have found correlation.

Further information on the diagnosis of PSCC can be found in Trowbridge & Walker's *The Yeast Syndrome*.[2] However, in terms of the deeper right *Chi* position, I read this as indicating a problem with the Large Intestine. This way of reading the pulse is based on Li Shi-zhen's system which historically has been supported by Li Shi-cai and later by Wu Qian, editor of the *Yi Zong Jin Jian* (*The Golden Mirror of the Medical*

Tradition), one of the late Qing Dynasty's most influential medical compendia. This method is theoretically based on the relationship of the Internal Duct of the Triple Heater with the Small and Large Intestines and the creation of Postnatal or Acquired Kidney Yin and Yang from the Pure of the Impure of Liquids and Foods respectively. This is somewhat abstruse and complicated theory but theory which I find clinically vital. This theory helps explain the crucial importance of healthy Large Intestine function, something contemporary TCM has largely overlooked.

Western naturopaths have emphasized the pivotal role in pathology of the colon for over a hundred years. Recently, Western researchers, such as Dr. Jeffrey Katke, clinical nutritionist, have stated that the large intestine is the basis of the immune system.[2] I believe this opinion is supported by TCM theory as well. The Large Intestine is the Root of the *Wei Qi* and Kidney Yang production which, on the one hand, protects the Surface from invasion, and, on the other, catalyzes the creation and transformation (*Sheng Hua*) of *Jing* Essence. In addition, the Large Intestine has a number of important reciprocal relationships with other Organs which effect the production and distribution of Postnatal or Acquired Qi and, therefore, Essence. These reciprocal relationships include the Large Intestine/Stomach, the Large Intestine/Lungs, the Large Intestine/Liver, the Large Intestine/Kidneys, and the Large Intestine and the *Bao Gong/Qi Hai Dan Tian*.

Many American TCM practitioners read a deep right *Chi* as a sign of Kidney Yang Deficiency. However, most often in young and middle-aged patients, such a reading is not corroborated by the other presenting signs and symptoms. Although the patient may be chronically fatigued, they more often have digestive and intestinal complaints. I typically see this scenario in patients with various viral infections, such as EBV, CMV, and HIV. When I come across this pulse sign in such patients,

I check the right *Guan* or Gate position. If it is superficially more prominent than the left *Guan* but then mushes out or becomes weak beneath, I read this as a weak Spleen, Hot Stomach, and Damp Heat in the Large Intestine. Most often these patients also have a floating, fine left *Chi* and a wiry pulse overall. This I read as an over-active Small Intestine with weak Kidney *Jing* and chronic Liver Qi.

In such cases, an over-active Stomach and Small Intestine coupled with a weak Spleen may give rise to polyuria without actual Kidney Qi Deficiency. This is complicated by Liver Qi causing Stagnation of the Large Intestine as well. Dampness percolates down from the Middle and becomes entangled with Heat arising from the Liver. This Damp Heat effects the Lower Burner as a whole but specifically can impact the Large Intestine if it is Stagnant as well. The right *Chi* is deep not because the Kidney Yang is weak *per se*. A deep pulse can simply mean an Internal disease, i.e. a disease which is flourishing within as opposed to on the Surface. The TCM definition of the Inside as opposed to the Outside is the *Zang Fu*. Dampness and Heat coupled with Stagnation impair the arisal of Clear Yang and, therefore, the pulse is deep.

To complete this frequently encountered pulse picture, the right *Cun*, which I read in women as the Heart tends to be somewhat weak and the left *Cun*, which I read in women as the Lungs, tends to be astringent superficially. This indicates to me a *Shen* Spirit unnourished and insecure or, in other words, anxious, and lingering Evil Heat in the Lungs causing bouts of otherwise unexplainable sadness and depression.

When I suspect that PSCC is complicating any of my viral patients, including those with CIN, I first administer a candidicidal regime. This consists initially of 2 weeks on Metagenics' Ultrabalance. This is a hypoallergenic, yeast-free, liquid meal replacement. This is mixed with vegetables juices, broth, skim milk, or plain water along with which the patient may eat fresh, steamed vegetables. This Ultrabalance program includes within it fiber bulking agents which aid in promoting bowel movements, thus expelling Turbidity and clearing Heat from the Large Intestine.

Along with this, I administer Health Concerns' Phellostatin. Phellostatin is a combination of Chinese herbs manufactured in tablet form designed to tonify and invigorate the Spleen and clear Heat and Dampness from all three Burners but especially from the Lower *Jiao*. Phellostatin's ingredients are:

>Cortex Phellodendri
>Rhizoma Anemarrhenae
>Herba Artemesiae Capillaris
>Radix Dioscoreae Oppositae
>Radix Codonopsis Pilosulae
>Semen Plantaginis
>Fructus Cnidii Monnieri
>Rhizoma Atractylodis
>Radix Pulsatillae Chinensis
>Herba Houttuyniae Cordatae
>Fructus Amomi Cardamomi
>Radix Glycyrrhizae

Of these ingredients, Phellodendron, Houttuynia, and Cnidium Monnierum have all demonstrated significant anti-fungal effects.[4] Whereas, Phellodendron and Pulsatilla have been shown to have pronounced anti-bacterial effect.[5] As Trowbridge and Walker in *The Yeast Syndrome* describe, often yeast and bacteria have a symbiotic relationship:

>If bacterial colonies are remaining in tissues after antibiotics are discontinued, safely shielded inside a colony of surrounding yeast, then only by killing the C. albicans at the same time

can a physician effectively eradicate all of the patient's bacterial organisms. It is the only way to rid his patient of the bacteria that would remain to seed the next infection in the following weeks or months.[6]

As a background or beverage tea, the patient is also allowed and even encouraged to drink an infusion or decoction of Pau D'Arco or Taheebo (Cortex Tabebuiae Impetiginosae). My TCM description of this famous South American herb is that it is Sweet, Acrid, and Neutral. It enters the Stomach/Spleen, Bladder, and Liver. It drains Dampness from the Lower Burner, facilitates the separation of Clear and Turbid, clears and eliminates Damp Heat from the skin, and dissolves Damp Toxins. Because it has anti-tumor properties, it probably also should be said to relieve swelling and combat cancer. Pau D'Arco is widely believed to be candidicidal.

During this phase of candida therapy, the emphasis is on *Qu Xie* or attacking Evil in the form of *Chong* (parasites) and Damp Heat. Also during this phase, some patients may experience aggravation of their symptoms. This is due to toxicity in turn due to the massive die-off of yeast. This is called in the candida literature a Herxheimer reaction. Although many clinicians hail it as a favorable sign indicating successful candidicide, it can be very uncomfortable and even intolerable to the patient. In such cases, the dosage of candidicidal medicinals should be reduced and coffee enemas or colonic lavage administered. Coffee enemas here are for the purpose of clearing Heat and eliminating Dampness, promoting bowel movements and the discharge of Turbidity, activating the Qi and Blood, promoting the arisal of Clear Yang, and dissipating Stagnation and Accumulation. Patients experiencing Herxheimer reactions should also drink more water and may do dry brushing and take Epsom salt baths. However, because Ultrabalance includes bulking agents which themselves promote healthy bowel function, Herxheimer reactions amongst my patients have been minimal.

After 2 weeks of such a candidicidal regime, I switch emphasis to *Fu Zheng* or supporting the Righteous. The patient is allowed to return to a moderately restrictive, yeast-free diet. They are encouraged to eat plenty of fresh, cooked vegetables, occasional meat and eggs, unrefined or partially refined grains, and limited amounts of fruits. They are encouraged to stay away from yeasted breads, fermented foods, alcohol, vinegar, dairy products, and concentrated sweets. See Appendix IV for a more complete list of dietary do's and don'ts during this phase. At the same time, they are given Metagenics' Ultrabifidus and Ultradophilus in rotation along with Probioplex and Azeopangen. All these nutritional supplements are for the purpose of encouraging normal, healthy Stomach/Spleen/Large Intestine function and digestion.

Ultrabifidus is made from live Bacteria Lactobacilli Bifidi, one of the healthy commensal bacteria which live in the intestine and keep Candida Albicans under control. We receive Bifidus bacteria with our mother's milk. Therefore, if a person has had antibiotics which kill Bifidus bacteria after having been weaned, they may have little way of restoring this intestinal flora. In addition, Bifidus bacteria populations decline with the aging process commensurate with the decline of *Jing* and the Kidneys.

Ultradophilus is made from live Bacteria Lactobacilli Acidophili, better known simply as Acidophilus. Acidophilus is the other important, healthy, commensal bacterium that helps keep Candida populations in check. When used in rotation, one takes 1 teaspoon of Ultrabifidus TID with meals until one bottle is finished. This is then followed by one bottle of Ultradophilus at 1/2 teaspoon TID. This regime is repeated at least 2 times or 2 bottles each of Ultrabifidus and Ultradophilus. Both these powders are made from patented strains of these bacteria guaranteed to survive the hydrochloric acid in the stomach and bile in the small intestine. They both must be kept refrigerated to maintain their potency and are taken mixed with tepid water to be drunk.

Probioplex, another Metagenics product, is a globulin concentrate made from whey. Enzyme-linked immuno-sorbent assay (ELISA) techniques have shown that whey contains viable antibodies to bacterial and viral pathogens and the toxins produced by these pathogens.[7] In particular, Probioplex has demonstrated antibody reactions against such common intestinal pathogens as E. Coli, Salmonella Dublin, and Haemophilus Saunus.[8] Probioplex is quite effective in helping to control loose stools and diarrhea in HIV-infected patients and in general promotes good bowel movements through the clearing and elimination of Damp Heat from the *Yang Ming*. 2 teaspoons are taken TID after meals mixed in room temperature water. It can be taken right along with either Ultradophilus or Ultrabifidus. It can be used until bowel movements are normal according to TCM parameters.

Azeopangen is the brand name for Metagenics' digestive enzymes which are taken with meals. Azeopangen is manufactured from raw pancreas concentrate and contains:

    Protease
    Amylase
    Lipase
    Peptidases
    Nucleases
    Elastases

From the TCM perspective, pancreatic digestive enzymes such as these tonify the Spleen and benefit the Qi. They promote ascension of the Clear and descension of the Turbid, thus harmonizing the Middle. In addition, researchers have found that pancreatic enzymes aid in restoring proper intestinal flora and in the nutritional management of gastrointestinal bacterial over-growth problems.[9] This also makes sense from a TCM perspective. Since it is the Spleen *Yun Hua* function which ascends the Clear and descends the Turbid, tonification and regulation of the Spleen does inhibit Dampness from percolating downward and Heat from accumulating in the Liver and Large Intestine. Azeopangen are taken with meals, 1-2 tablets per meal.

The use of digestive enzymes and bacterial replacement therapy has its classical precedent in Chinese medicine. Massa Medica Fermentata (Shen Qu) is a fermented herbal product which essentially contains bacteria and digestive enzymes. Shen Qu is categorized as a Stagnant Food dispersing medicinal in TCM which benefits the digestion and harmonizes the Stomach. Its use is indicated diagnostically in part by a thick, greasy tongue coating which, as thrush, is also indicative of a yeast overgrowth.

Usually during this phase of anti-candida treatment, concomitant Chinese herbal therapy can be initiated for the rectification of any TCM menopathies as can acupuncture and topical treatments to the cervix and vagina. Although PSCC or polysystemic chronic candidiasis is not a traditional Chinese disease category, in my experience, it is an important complicating condition which should be dealt with first. If not, it can lead both practitioner and patient around and around chasing ever-shifting, ever-recurring signs and symptoms without achieving any sense of meaningful progress.

As mentioned above, I see no conceptual or theoretical reason why candidiasis cannot be added to the "Chinese" disease categories under the heading *Chong* or parasites. When such a diagnosis is made, the requisite therapeutic principle is to *Sha*

Jun or kill yeast. In modern Chinese TCM, *Sha Jun* means to kill microbes. When used as a descriptive of a medicine's properties, these words are usually translated as anti-microbial. However, in the case of candidiasis, its more literal translation is even more appropriate and technically descriptive.

AMOEBIASIS

A similar and often concomitantly complicating condition is amoebiasis. Various protozoans may also parasitize the intestines causing dysbiosis and indigestion. According to TCM, such protozoans are not usually classified as *Chong* and the problems they cause are usually treated under the Patterns Spleen Qi Deficiency, Spleen Dampness, and Damp Heat. Although I think TCM generally treats amoebiasis better than it treats candidiasis, still it is also possible that a more conscious and deliberate inclusion of this category of parasitosis and, therefore, even more conscious and deliberate treatment for it is warranted by current research and state-of-the-art environmental medicine.

Recently researchers have shown that amoebiasis, principally giardiasis, accompanies many cases of CFIDS (Chronic Fatigue Immune Deficiency Syndrome) and many cases of chronic indigestion. Often these two disease categories overlap, with most CFIDS patients also suffering from some sort of digestive disturbance. These patients may have loose stools, constipation, or alternating constipation and diarrhea. In addition, they often complain of flatulence and abdominal distention after eating. Treatment aimed at eliminating pathogenic amoebae has been shown to be effective in the treatment of both CFIDS and chronic digestive complaints.[10]

Diagnosis of amoebiasis in Western environmental medicine is mostly made by microscopic inspection of the stools or rectal mucosa. Besides microscopy, it can also be diagnosed by Vega biokinesiology (VBK). The same pulse pattern described above of a deeper right *Chi* may also be indicative of amoebiasis for essentially the same reasons. Since many patients have both yeast and protozoans simultaneously, their distinction *vis a vis* the pulse may be moot. It is my opinion that patients' with chronic viral infections and digestive difficulties who do not respond adequately to the above anti-candida regime should be tried on an anti-amoebiasis regime.

The anti-amoebiasis regime I employ is based on the use of Health Concerns' Aquilaria 22. This is a 22 ingredient herbal tablet whose composition is based on both Chinese and Tibetan medical theory. It is meant to tonify the Spleen and benefit the Qi, eliminate Dampness both by transportation and transformation, to clear Heat and disperse Turbidity downward, and the expel *Chong* or parasites. Its indications are chronic indigestion due to parasitosis and dysbiosis of the intestines. Its ingredients are:

> Lignum Aquilariae Agallochae
> Rhizoma Recens Zingiberis
> Fructus Pruni Mume
> Radix Codonopsis Pilosulae
> Fructus Terminaliae Chebulae
> Sclerotium Poriae Cocoris
> Rhizoma Atractylodis Macrocephalae
> Fructus Quisqualis Indicae
> Fructificatio Polypori Mylittae
> Radix Saussureae Seu Vladmiriae
> Semen Torreyae Grandis
> Semen Arecae Catechu
> Pericarpium Punicae Granati
> Cortex Meliae Azerdach
> Radix Rubiae Cordifoliae
> Fructus Citri Seu Ponciri

Fructus Myristicae Fragrantis
Fructus Amomi Cardamomi
Pasta Ulmi Macrocarpi
Fructus Zanthoxyli Bungeani
Radix Glycyrrhizae
Extractum Dessicatum Herbae Aloes

Codonopsis, Poria, and Atractylodes tonify the Spleen and benefit the Qi in addition to transporting and transforming Liquids. Saussurea regulates the Qi and helps harmonize Liver Wood with Spleen Qi. In both Chinese and Tibetan medicines, Saussurea is used for abdominal distention. It has a special tropism for the Lower Burner and the Large Intestine in particular. Ginger harmonizes the Stomach and transforms Dampness and Turbidity. It helps regulate ascension and descension. Licorice tonifies the Qi, especially of the Heart, but in this formula is primarily meant to moderate and soften the effects of the numerous, somewhat harsh ingredients. The other ingredients are not so well known or so commonly used and, therefore, merit individual description.

Lignum Aquilariae Agallochae (Aquilaria) is one of the most important Ayurvedic and Tibetan medicinal ingredients. In those medicines, it is used as the main ingredient to regulate the Qi *vis a vis* the mind and emotions. Specifically in Tibetan medicine, Aquilaria is used to clear Heat from the Heart. In TCM, Aquilaria is a *Li Qi* medicinal. It moves the Qi, stops pain, reverses Rebellion, directs the Qi downwards, and aids in the Kidneys' grasping the Qi. This implies that it harmonizes the Lungs and Kidneys and, therefore, further implies an influence on the Large Intestine both through *Yin Yang/Biao Li* and Internal Gate theories. Based on both Chinese and Tibetan usage, I believe we can say Aquilaria redirects *Ming Men* Fire back down to its Root in the Kidneys.

Fructus Pruni Mume (Mume) is an astringent medicinal. It

contains leakage of Lung Qi, stops cough, restrains leakage from the Intestines, stops diarrhea, generates Fluids, expels Worms (specifically roundworms), stops bleeding, and alleviates thirst. Astringency of the Lower Burner is dominated by the Kidney Qi. Therefore, Mume has a relationship with the Lungs and the Kidneys, the Lungs and the Large Intestine, and the Large Intestine and the Kidneys. It is a specific for dysbiosis of the bowels.

Fructus Terminaliae Chebulae (Myrobalan) is another very famous Ayurvedic and Tibetan medicinal. In TCM, it is used in fairly large doses (9-12 g p.d.) and is used to stop diarrhea and astringe the Intestines. In Ayurveda, it is used, as in this tablet, in smaller doses as a nutritive purgative. Like Mume above, Myrobalan works on harmonizing the Lungs and Large Intestine and the Lung Qi's empowerment of Large Intestine function. In Tibetan medicine, Myrobalan is also used to treat Lung diseases and to reduce Excess Bile. This implies a relationship between the Lungs, Large Intestine, and Liver which I believe is of utmost clinical importance.

Fructus Quisqualis Indicae (Quisqualis), as its pharmacological name suggests, is probably originally an Indian herb. It is a Worm-expelling medicinal which kills Worms and strengthens the Spleen at the same time as it disperses Accumulations.

Fructificatio Polypori Mylittae (Omphalia) also kills Worms. As does Semen Torryae Grandis (Torreya). Other *Qu Chong* ingredients include Semen Arecae Catechu (Areca or Betelnut) which kills Worms, drains downwards, leads out Stagnation, moves the Qi, and promotes urination, and Cortex Meliae Azerdach (Melia) which kills Worms and also treats vaginal trichomoniasis. In Tibetan medicine, it is believed that Areca is good for the Kidneys. This again underscores the relationship between the Large Intestine and the Kidneys which I find so important in my clinical practice.

Pericarpium Punicae Granati (Pomegranate), like Mume and Myrobalan, is an astringent. It restrains leakage from the Intestines and stops diarrhea. It also kills Worms. As a *Sha Jun* or anti-microbial agent, Pomegranate kills various species of bacteria, fungi, and viruses as well as intestinal amoebae. In Tibetan medicine, Pomegranate reduces Phlegm. This suggests that it, like so many other *Qu Chong* ingredients discussed herein, has a definite effect on the Lungs, the storehouse of Phlegm, and further underscores the Lungs and Large Intestine's *Biao Li* relationship.

Radix Rubiae Cordifoliae (Rubia) cools the Blood, stops bleeding, promotes the circulation of Blood, and disperses Stagnant Blood. Its Chinese and Tibetan use is quite similar. Tibetan doctors say Rubia is for fever due to traumatic injury resulting in extravasation and Stagnation. Rubia has also demonstrated antibiotic and anti-viral effects *in vitro*.

Fructus Citri Seu Ponciri (Chih-shih or Aurantium) is a *Li Qi* medicinal which cracks or breaks up Stagnant Qi. It reduces Accumulations, directs the Qi downward, and moves the stool. Actually, in this formula, this ingredient should be written as Fructus Immaturus Citri Seu Ponciri (Chih-ko, Chi Ke) since it more specifically than the mature fruit effects the Lower Burner and moves the stool. However, in modern TCM, many practitioners no longer make this distinction.

Fructus Myristicae Fragrantis (Nutmeg) is also an astringent. It restrains leakage from the Intestines and stops diarrhea. It warms the Middle, moves the Qi, and stops pain. However, in Tibetan medicine, Nutmeg specifically is used to regulate the *Ming Men* Fire and to redirect it down from the Heart back to the Kidneys. It is believed to have a pronounced regularizing effect on the Heart Spirit and is one of the man ingredients in Tibetan medicine for treating psychoemotional disturbances. In Korean medicine, it is said that a small amount of Nutmeg makes almost any formula work faster.[11]

Fructus Amomi Cardamomi (Cardomom) invigorates the Spleen, aromatically transforms Dampness, warms the Middle, moves the Qi and transforms Stagnation. It is one of the Six Great Medicines of Buddhism and is specific for the Spleen.

Pasta Ulmi Macrocarpi (Ulmus) kills Worms. It is anti-fungal, killing many species of yeast.

Fructus Zanthoxyli Bungeani (Zanthoxylum or Szechuan Pepper) warms the Middle, alleviates pain, disperses Cold, and kills Worms. In Tibetan medicine, it is believed to "open" the Channels to allow deep penetration of other medicinals into areas that otherwise might not be reached. This is based on the ability of aromatic substances to penetrate and permeate Yin.

Extractum Dessicatum Herbae Aloes (Dried Aloe Vera Juice) is a Cold purgative. It enters both the Liver and Large Intestine clearing Heat from both. We will have more to say about this ingredient below.

For amoebiasis and dysbiosis of the Large Intestine, this formula can be taken for several weeks. I have found this formula quite effective in my clinical practice. Its theoretical basis is profound and well-knit. Yet the proof of its excellence is in its empirical efficacy.

HERPES GENITALIA

Herpes simplex virus II, better known as herpes genitalia, is a common concurrent infection in women with CIN. Several years ago, researchers felt HSV II was the main etiological factor in cervical dysplasia/cervical cancer. More recently, attention and blame has been shifted to HPV or human papilloma virus as the Western medical microbial pathogen. The exact inter-relationship between HPV, HSV II, and CIN is not clear. It is probable that there is some synergistic potentiation between these two viruses. At the very least, HSV II is essentially the same kind of pathogen as HPV according to TCM -- a Warm Hidden Evil lying latent in the *Xue Fen* or Blood Phase of the Foot *Jue Yin*.

When HSV II goes from latent to active, it takes some time to move from deep within the body to the Surface. As it does so, it causes trauma or injury to the internal tissue before it erupts on the Exterior. Drs. Eric R. Braverman and Carl C. Pfeiffer, in *The Healing Nutrients Within*, describe this in terms of Western medicine:

> When a patient recovers from the primary herpes simplex viral infection, the virus settles in the nearby nerves and spinal ganglia, where it is protected from circulatory antibodies. Because herpes reactivation and growth always begins in the ganglion cells, every case of recurrent herpes simplex viral infection is a ganglionitis. The virus then passes down the nerves to induce the formation of the herpetic blister in the skin or mucous membranes, but this represents only the 'rim of the volcano'. This means that every time a person has a cold sore on his or her lip, the base of the brain, where the cranial nerve's exit, may also be involved. Herpes simplex may be considered a chronic disease of the nerves which periodically spreads to the skin.[12]

Although the preceding paragraph primarily describes the course of herpes simplex I, the same thing can be said about herpes simplex II and even herpes zoster. In the case of HSV II, the virus remains latent in the sacral ganglia from which it moves out and along the nerves on its way to the genitalia in an acute outbreak. However, the virus does not necessarily always progress to the Surface of the body, but can go from latent to active and cause inflammation of the tissue and nerves it passes through without resulting in superficial lesions. Therefore, a number of medical complaints in infected patients may, in fact, be due to active inflammation by the herpes virus without skin lesions. The following is a list compiled by Braverman and Pfeiffer of the possible diseases caused by HSV I & II.[13]

Skin Diseases

Vesicular skin eruptions
Eczema herpeticum (Kaposi's varicelliform eruption)
Traumatic herpes (herpes gladiatorum secondary to burns)
Herpetic whitlow

Mucous Membrane Diseases

Acute gingivostomatitis
Recurrent stomatitis
Cervicitis

Mucocutaneous Junction Diseases

Herpes labialis (fever blisters)
Herpes progenitalis
Vulvovaginitis

Eye Diseases

Conjunctivitis
Keratoconjunctivitis

Central Nervous System Diseases

Meningoencephalitis
Myelitis
Radiculitis
Trigeminal neuralgia
Tic douloureux
Bell's palsy

Systemic Infections

Acute respiratory diseases
Tracheobronchitis
Pneumonia
Disseminated disease of the newborn
Hepatitis
Cystitis

Hypersensitivity Reactions

Erythema multiforme

Malignancies

Cervical and oral cancer

This movement from within to without is, in a sense, retrograde when compared to the normal progression of a *Wen Xie* or Warm Evil. However, it is characteristic of so many of our modern viral diseases.

Although the therapy for HPV and cervical dysplasia outlined above so far does have an ameliorating effect on HSV II, still, it is my belief that flare-ups of herpes genitalia should be dealt with specifically and aggressively since I cannot help but believe that if this Damp Heat Toxin is active on the Outside, HPV is simultaneously and synergistically flourishing on the Inside.

Astra Isatis

Often herpes attacks or outbreaks are preceded by prodromal signs and symptoms. These, in fact, are the evidence that Evil Qi is active within causing Internal Injury. When there are prodromal or premonitory signs and symptoms, there are several Chinese formulas which are effective for aborting the attack and returning the Evil Qi to its relatively latent or Hidden state. The first of these is Health Concerns' Astra Isatis. The ingredients in this tableted formula are:

>Radix Isatidis
>Radix Astragali Seu Hedysari
>Radix Bupleuri
>Thallus Algae
>Radix Codonopsis Pilosulae
>Fructus Lycii
>Radix Dioscoreae Oppositae
>Herba Epimedii
>Fructus Broussonetiae
>Rhizoma Atractylodis
>Radix Glycyrrhizae

Essentially, this formula tonifies Kidney *Jing* while at the same time clearing Heat, eliminating Dampness, and dissolving Toxins. Astragalus, Codonopsis, and Dioscorea tonify the Qi. Lycium tonifies the Liver Blood and Kidney Yin, thus benefitting *Jing* Essence. Fructus Broussonetiae does likewise. It is my opinion that both of these ingredients also quell Deficient Yin Fire (although the barks of both may be more effective for specifically this purpose). Broussonetia has a special tropism for the genitalia and an alterative effect on genital fluxes and venereal diseases. Epimedium tonifies both Yin and Yang at the same time as it harnesses Ascendant Liver Yang and disperses it. Rhizoma Atractylodis invigorates the Spleen and transforms Dampness in the Middle Burner while it seeps Dampness from the Lower Burner. Bupleurum dredges Liver Qi and relieves constraint, remembering that the Foot *Jue Yin* irrigates the genitalia. Thallus Algae, aka Laminaria, scatters Phlegm Nodulation and, at first, may seem out of place in this formula. However, classically, Laminaria was used to treat *Shan Bing* or diseases in men of the genitalia and groin. This class of disease includes seven subcategories, at least one of which is identical to Damp Heat. Laminaria relieves swelling and has a known, traditional tropism for the lower half of the body. If taken at 2 1/2 times the normal recommended dose or 8 pills TID, Astra Isatis can help abort a herpes outbreak.

Qi Wu Jiang Xia Tang

Another formula which can be effective for aborting herpes outbreaks for those who experience prodromal signs and symptoms before the appearance of skin lesions is Qi Wu Jiang Xia Tang. This is available as a desiccated extract from Qualiherbs under the name Tang Kuei & Gambir Combination. *Qi Wu* means seven ingredients. *Jiang Xia* means blood pressure lowering. *Tang* means decoction. This formula was created by Otsuka Keisetsu to treat hypertension in middle-aged men. Its ingredients are:

Radix Angelicae Sinensis
Radix Paeoniae Albae
Radix Rehmanniae
Radix Ligustici Chuanxiong
Radix Astragali Seu Hedysari
Ramulus Uncariae Cum Uncis
Cortex Phellodendri

Practitioners will recognize the first four ingredients as Si Wu Tang, the four ingredients for tonifying the Blood. However, these four ingredients also tonify the *Jing* as well due to the close relationship between the *Jing* and the Blood. Astragalus tonifies the Qi and promotes the *Sheng Hua* or creation of Blood and Essence. Ramulus Uncariae Cum Uncis, aka Gambir, extinguishes Wind but also clears Heat from the Liver. Phellodendron clears and eliminates Damp Heat from the Lower Burner. In the treatment of hypertension, this formula is meant to treat Internal Stirring of Wind due to Liver Blood Deficiency with a tendency to Hyperactive *Ming Men Huo*. However, because it benefits *Jing* Essence, clears Heat from the Liver, and eliminates Dampness from the Lower Burner, it can also forestall a herpes outbreak which has just begun internally. This formula is particularly effective if the prodromal symptom is sacral and sciatic pain due to Gambir's extinguishing Wind and this being a Windy kind of pain.

Bioradiance

Bioradiance is a Western herbal tincture created by an eccentric millionaire in the Rocky Mountain West. It has been used clandestinely to treat a wide range of recalcitrant diseases both in humans and animals. In humans, it has been used with reported clinical success for the treatment of various cancers, various viral diseases, including HSV II, HPV, and HIV, and candidiasis. In animals, it has been used to treat bovine leukemia which is of known viral origin. This tincture is being distributed as an experimental medicine by K'an Herbs to TCM practitioners for the treatment of herpes and HIV. Although Bioradiance is a *Mi Fang* or secret formula in that its creator and manufacturer will not disclose the precise method of its preparation, its ingredients are known and, therefore, a tentative TCM description of its functions may be made. Its listed ingredients are:

    Radix Et Rhizoma Gentianae Campestris
    Rhizoma Sanguinariae Canadensis
    Herba Cum Radice Impatientis Pallidae
    Rhizoma Hydrastis Canadensis
    Gummum Galbani
    Herba Fumariae Officinalis
    Radix Fraserae Carolinensis
    Allicin

These ingredients are extracted in liquid Chlorophyll and combined with a number of minerals. According to this formula's creator, who wishes to remain anonymous, these minerals help create the proper electrical charge, thus providing the tropism for this medicinal to enter diseased cells.

Two of the herbal ingredients in this formula are species of the family Gentianaceae. The first is Radix Et Rhizoma Gentianae Campestris. It is Bitter and Cold and enters the Liver and Gallbladder. It clears Heat and eliminates Dampness, relieves depression and constraint, clears Liver Fire, clears Heat and dissolves Toxins, and harmonizes Wood and Earth.

Radix Fraserae Carolinensis is also called American Colombo. It differs from the Tibetan medicinal Swertia Chirata botanically only by the presence of a style. Swertia is used in Tibetan medicine to clear Heat from the Liver/Gallbladder. Similarly, Frasera is Bitter and Cool. It clears Heat and eliminates Dampness from the Liver/Gallbladder. It also clears Heat from the Stomach and Intestines and promotes bowel movements. Because it clears Heat from the Stomach, it is also useful for the treatment of vomiting and nausea due to Heat. Colombo enters the Liver, Gallbladder, Stomach, and Large Intestine Channels and harmonizes the *Shao Yang Fen.* Lloyd Brothers, Pharmacists, Inc. of Cincinnati, a famous Eclectic herbal medicinal manufacturer at the turn of the century, marketed a Colloidum Frasera as a remedy for atonic constipation, i.e. constipation due to lack of peristalsis. This suggests once again the Liver's relationship with the Large Intestine and *vice versa.*

Rhizoma Sanguinariae Canadensis or simply Sanguinaria is Acrid, Bitter, and Hot. It enters the Liver, Lungs, Stomach, and Spleen. It should probably be categorized like Evodia as an Interior-warming, Cold-dispelling medicinal. It dispels Cold, stops pain, and stops vomiting. It is used for Liver/Stomach Channel Cold Phlegm disorders. It redirects Rebellious Qi downward and stops vomiting due to disharmony of the Liver/Stomach. Because it redirects Rebellious Qi downward and transforms Phlegm, it is also used for Lung Heat and Liver/Lung cough. Further, Sanguinaria combats cancer. When combined with Hydrastis, its use is similar to combining Evodia with Coptis.

Herba Cum Radice Impatientis Pallidae is Jewelweed. It is Sweet, Neutral, Cool, and Toxic. It enters the Spleen and Lungs. It expels Water by purging downward, clears Heat and reduces swelling, and relieves swelling and dissipates Nodulations. It is essentially a harsh cathartic.

Rhizoma Hyrastis Canadensis is Goldenseal. It is Bitter and Cold and enters the Heart, Liver, Stomach, and Large Intestine. It purges Fire and dissolves Toxins, clears Heat and eliminates Dampness, drains Stomach Fire, and clears Heat from the Surface topically.

Gummum Galbani is an aromatic resin derived from Ferula Galbaniflua. G.A. Stuart[14] and Hong-yen Hsu et al.[15] identify this as Asafoetida. Asafoetida is Acrid and Warm and enters the Stomach and Spleen Channels. It disperses Food Stagnation, particularly due to over-consumption of meat. It conducts Qi downward, disperses Stagnations and Accumulations, and kills Chong. It is used for the treatment of intestinal parasites, abdominal swelling, Cold pain in the Heart and abdomen, distention and pain in the chest and abdomen, and dysentery.

Herba Fumariae Officinalis, aka Fumitory, is Bitter and Cool and enters the Liver, Gallbladder, Stomach, and Large Intestine. Fumitory purges Heat and moves the stool, clears and eliminates Damp Heat, clears Heat and dissolves Toxins, and invigorates the Blood and cracks Congealed Blood.

Allicin is one of the active ingredients in Bulbus Alli Sativi or Garlic. Garlic is categorized in TCM as a parasite-expelling/killing medicinal. It is Acrid and Warm. Its TCM functions are that it kills parasites and dissolves Toxins, here mostly meaning Fire Toxins of the Intestines. In TCM, preparations of Garlic are used to treat pinworms, amoebiasis, bacillary dysentery, mycoses, and fungi. Laboratory tests and folk beliefs, both Western and Oriental, suggest Garlic has a *Kang Ai* or cancer-combatting effect *vis a vis* breast and liver cancers. Allicin has a strong but variable antibiotic effect. Garlic is both Warm and a *Jie Du* or Toxin-dissolving medicinal. This helps dispel the common but not totally accurate perception that all *Jie Du* medicinals are Cold.

Chlorophyll is Sweet, slightly Salty, Astringent, and Neutral. It is nutritive in that it tonifies the Qi and Blood. However, it also clears Heat, dissolves Toxins, and generates New Tissue. Modern Western use also suggests it has a *Kang Ai* or cancer-combatting effect.

Bioradiance is similar to several other formulas in Chinese medicine which each address all Six Stagnations. Ping Xiao Dan is somewhat similar. Yue Qu Wan (Stagnation Dispelling Pill) is another formula which contains ingredients for Food, Phlegm, Heat, Dampness, Qi, and Blood Stagnations. The difference between Bioradiance and these Chinese formulas is that each of this formula's ingredients is also either *Jie Du* (Toxin-dissolving), *Qu Chong* (parasite-expelling), or *Sha Jun* (microbe-killing).

So far, I have had some success with treating persons with HIV and HSV II with Bioradiance. Although it is expensive for an as yet experimental formula, when CIN patients also suffer from frequent, repeated herpes outbreaks, I think this formula should be tried. This is especially the case in women whose herpes attacks have not responded to other, more conventional formulas or therapy. Preliminary reports suggest that this formula will put an end to recurrent outbreaks of herpes within 6 weeks to 3 months of initiating therapy. Patients who, prior to initiating treatment with Bioradiance, had herpes outbreaks once or twice a month for years have gone a year without further recurrence.[16] To date, my own clinical experience with this formula substantiates these reports.

When treating herpes genitalia with Bioradiance, the recommended protocol is 3 drops TID for the first ounce (i.e. 66 days), 2 drops TID for the second ounce (i.e. 100 days), and 1 drop TID for the third ounce (i.e. 200 days). After one year of treatment, patients can either discontinue the Bioradiance entirely or take a maintenance dose of 1 drop per day. The creator of Bioradiance feels that it can eliminate HPV as well as HSV I & II, in which case cessation of herpes outbreaks may indicate that the HPV has also been neutralized. Since it is difficult to asses the status of latent HPV in asymptomatic individuals, use of Bioradiance in such women may be an expensive gamble. However, in those with active HSV II, this expense seems warranted, since it has demonstrated effectiveness in neutralizing that virus at least.

Many textbooks suggest the use of Long Dan Xie Gan Tang (Dragon Gall Liver Purging Decoction) for the treatment of an acute attack of herpes genitalia. For instance, *A Handbook of Traditional Chinese Dermatology* lists this formula for the treatment of *Nu Yin Kuei Yang* (Ulceration of the Female Genitalia).[17] Such vaginal ulcers are divided into two types in TCM dermatology: the gangrenous variety and the venereal variety. The venereal variety are characterized as shallow ulcers with some pain but generally few if any systemic symptoms. However, there is nodular erythema. This description covers herpes genitalia. Long Dan Xie Gan Tang is for the purgation of Liver Fire and Damp Heat from the Liver/Gallbladder and Lower Burner. It is a good treatment if the patient is simply Excess, but, in my experience, it does not work so well in women whose conditions are more typically Combined Excess/Deficiency Patterns. When this formula is used, it should only be used for relatively short periods of time during the most acute phase. Long Dan Xie Gan Tang is available in tablet form as Quell Fire from K'an Herbs. Its ingredients are:

> Radix Gentianae Scabrae
> Radix Scutellariae Baicalensis
> Fructus Gardeniae
> Rhizoma Alismatis
> Semen Plantaginis
> Caulis Akebiae Mutong
> Radix Rehmanniae
> Apex Radicis Angelicae Sinensis
> Radix Bupleuri
> Radix Glycyrrhizae

Health Concerns also markets two other formulas in tablet

form which are useful for treating acute episodes of herpes genitalia. These are Coptis Purge Fire Tablets and Isatis Cooling Formula.

Coptis Purge Fire Tablets

    Rhizoma Coptidis
    Rhizoma Anemarrheane
    Radix Bupleuri
    Fructus Forsythiae
    Fructus Gardeniae
    Radix Scutellariae Baicalensis
    Cortex Phellodendri
    Radix Gentianae Scabrae
    Radix Paeoniae Rubrae
    Caulis Akebiae Mutong
    Radix Rehmanniae
    Herba Lophatheri Gracilis
    Radix Sophorae Flavescentis
    Radix Angelicae Sinensis
    Radix Glycyrrhizae

This formula clears Heat, eliminates Dampness, and dissolves Toxins. The addition of Bupleurum helps direct these ingredients to the Liver Channel. Although the formula can clear Heat from either the Upper or Lower Burners, I find it especially effective for treating Damp Hot Toxic skin lesions of the Lower Burner.

Isatis Cooling Formula

Isatis Cooling Formula is also for clearing Damp Heat Toxins from the Lower Burner. Its ingredients are:

    Extractum Herbae Cum Radice Isatidis
    Radix Bupleuri

Cortex Radicis Moutan
Radix Paeoniae Rubrae
Radix Codonopsis Pilosulae
Rhizoma Smilacis Glabrae
Radix Angelicae Sinensis
Rhizoma Alismatis
Concha Ostreae
Fructus Gardeniae
Caulis Akebiae Mutong
Rhizoma Cyperi

This formula, in addition to clearing Heat, eliminating Dampness, and dissolving Toxins, activates the Qi and Blood to disperse Stagnation. Isatis has anti-viral activity, while Smilax specifically treats venereal fluxes. The addition of Codonopsis is intended to strength the Stomach/Spleen against the Cold and attacking properties of the other ingredients thus protecting the *Zheng Qi*.

In addition to taking these or other similar formulas internally during acute herpes outbreaks, if there are wet, glistening lesions which are reluctant to scab and heal, one can mix a small amount of Realgar powder with isopropyl alcohol and apply this directly on the open part of the lesion. This should be repeated several times per day, but only on open, wet lesions, taking care not to get this orange "paint" on the surrounding tissue which it will tend to irritate. Typically, this will catalyze scabbing within 12-24 hours.

Also, acupuncture can and probably should be administered daily during a herpes outbreak. If initiated at the very first sign of an outbreak, it can sometimes abort the attack. At the least, acupuncture can make the discomfort less and hasten recovery. Usually I needle San Yin Jiao (Sp 6), Xue Hai (Sp 10), Xing Jian (Liv 2), Qu Quan (Liv 8), Yin Ling Quan (Sp 9), Yin Gu (Ki 10), and Hui Yin (CV 1). There is also an

Extra point called Yu Men Jiang (Jade Gate Pea) located slightly above the vaginal meatus. It is needled obliquely 0.3 *Cun* for skin diseases of the vagina. If lesions are further back on the sides of the labia, Extra point Ti Gang Ji (Lift Anus Muscle) can be needled unilaterally on the effected side. This point is located on the lateral edge of the vaginal orifice at the medial border of the labia majora towards the anus. For years I stayed away from points such as Hui Yin and Yu Men Jiang for modesty's sake. However, in the last two years, I have found that these points are simply the most effective local points for recurrent or recalcitrant vaginal lesions.

Another treatment for an acute genital herpes outbreak is fumigation. Fumigation or *Yan Yun Liao Fa* is a classical external treatment for dermatological lesions. Dr. (Eric) Tao Xi-yu, my first acupuncture teacher, has women stand over a lit moxa stick. In this case it is the moxa smoke directed to the lesion which is specifically therapeutic, not the heat. The moxa stick should be held far enough below the genitalia so that this therapy is *Yan Yun Liao Fa* and not *Wen Fa* or warming. The benefit of this treatment is that it can be done by the patient at home and does not require an office visit.

Intensive treatment with internal and externally administered herbs and acupuncture during an active herpes outbreak is meant to negate as much of the Evil Qi as possible. During its latent or hidden phase, the herpes virus is relatively impervious to the immune system. However, when this *Fu Wen Xie* is out and about, it can be attacked by the Righteous Qi. Treatment then is meant to reduce the virulence of the Evil Qi and not just to drive it back into its latent state.

CHAPTER FIVE
THE PREVENTIVE TREATMENT OF CIN DURING REMISSION

Because CIN is, in part, a viral disease, it is difficult to say that a patient has been cured just because they get one or several negative Paps. Although there are ViraPap tests which can detect the presence of invisible subclinical HPV, because Western medicine has no way to treat such invisible subclinical HPV, these tests are not routinely administered. In addition, they tend to be expensive. Therefore, at this writing, I can point to no patients who have tested positive for HPV, received the remedial treatment outlined above and gotten a good Pap, and who now test negative for HPV. Even though this may be possible, yet my current experience does not support this. I have only begun to experiment with homeopathic and potentized resonance filters and Vega biokinesiological testing (VBK) attempting to diagnose HPV in its latent or asymptomatic phase. When a Warm Evil goes hidden, it can remain so for years and even decades, silently stressing the immune system and causing occult inflammation and trauma, before it becomes obviously active. Therefore, the therapies I suggest for keeping both HPV and HSV II latent are similar to those used in their remedial treatment. However, the emphasis is even more on the Three Free Therapies, management of sex, lower doses of both herbal medicines and orthomolecular supplements, experimental use of modern, compound homotoxicological remedies, and a great deal of attention to maintaining healthy Large Intestine function.

DIET

The diet recommended during the remedial treatment of CIN is also the diet I recommend preventively as well. This is the healthy diet for the vast majority of Americans living in a temperate climate. This diet minimizes the accumulation of Dampness and Heat while maximizing the Postnatal production of Qi and Blood and, therefore, *Jing*.

The modern American diet is not the diet the human body evolved on over tens of millions of years. Our modern diet is based on interstate and intercontinental transportation, refrigeration, chemical preservation, and methods of preparation which all date from the last 50-70 years. Much before the Second World War, the average American did not have access to frozen foods, fruit juices, and raw salads year round. Prior to 120 years ago we did not have access to refined flour products. And prior to 200 years ago we did not have access to sugar. So many of the foods we take for granted as part of our modern diet are not even a blink on the evolutionary scale in terms of human nutritional history.

Our bodies evolved on grains, vegetables, and small amounts of animal protein. For hundreds of thousands of years, humans have cooked their food to make it more easily digestible. *Everything that we eat must be transformed into 100 degree soup in the Stomach before it can be assimilated.* Therefore, cooking food makes it more digestible and, consequently, more nutritious. Eating and drinking chilled, cold, and frozen foods may be relatively harmless when taken away from other meals, but, when eaten with other foods, these slow down and impede the digestion of anything else eaten at the same time. This is an extremely important point.

Even a little sugar is a lot considering that humans living in temperate climates historically almost never had access to such concentrated sweets. The average American today eats pounds of sugar per year. Likewise, we now consume pounds of preservatives and other chemicals which the human organism has never before been required to metabolize. Although it is a wonder that the human organism is as adaptive as it is, these are not optimal foods for living a healthy life.

The healthy diet for the vast majority of Americans living in temperate regions is one composed of complex carbohydrates, plenty of fresh, organically grown, lightly cooked vegetables, lots of fiber, small, occasional amounts of animal protein, occasional fruits and nuts, few sugars, not much oil, and as few chemicals as possible. By small, occasional amounts of animal protein, I mean not more than 2-3 oz. of meat per serving perhaps 3 times per week. This could be described as a Pritikin or Macrobiotic diet, but, whatever the name, it is the diet our bodies evolved on and the one on which our bodies thrive.

Although we may all have become habituated to our modern confections and delicacies, at best, these should be infrequent indulgences. The fact that we crave sugars, fats, spices, stimulants such as coffee and alcohol, and frozen treats such as ice cream in no way mitigates the fact that these foods are unhealthy. If eaten regularly, they result in disease. Therefore, I recommend all my patients to reflect back on the diet of their great, great grandparents and consider that as a model for themselves with the addition year round of more freshly cooked vegetables.

COLON CLEANSING

Since the Large Intestine is so vitally important in the maintenance of healthy Kidney function and consequently the function of the entire Triple Heater, I believe it is wise to pay special attention to this Bowel. Therefore, I often recommend a course of "colon cleansing" as one of the next steps after having received a negative Pap. If the patient has already been treated for candidiasis and/or parasitosis of the bowel and their bowel movements and intestinal function are fine, this treatment is usually not necessary. However, if previously little or no attention has been focused on the bowels, almost everyone can profit by a course of colon cleansing.

There are a number of possible regimes for promoting the healthy functioning of the Large Intestine. Colon cleansing is a Western naturopathic term and here the word cleansing does not imply clearing Heat as it does in its strict TCM usage. However, from a TCM point of view, we can think of colon cleansing as basically promoting the excretion of Turbid waste so that the Clear can all the better ascend. In our clinic, we use the Yerba Prima Internal Cleansing Program marketed by Yerba Prima Botanicals of Oakland, CA.

The Yerba Prima Internal Cleansing Program as we apply it consists of three adjuncts to the daily diet. These are:

> Kalenite Herbal Formula
> Colon Care Formula
> Aloe Vera Plus Herbs (or Oxy Toddy distributed by Eagle Marketing)

The Kalenite Herbal Formula consists of eight herbs. Although these are mostly Western herbs, their TCM functions are all appropriate for the regulation of the Large Intestine and Lower Burner. The ingredients in this formula are:

> Gummum Acaciae
> Folium Plantaginis

Herba Cardui Benedicti
Flos Caryophylli
Flos Trifolii
Radix Rumicis
Cortex Juglandis Cinerae

Aciacia Gum's TCM functions are essentially the same as Acacia Catechu's. It drains Dampness and absorbs seepage, stops bleeding, and arrests diarrhea. When used internally, Acacia primarily seeps Dampness from the Lower Burner and, in particular, from the Large Intestine.

Folium Plantaginis (Plantain Leaf) is Salty, Bitter, and Cold and enters the Lungs, Large Intestine, and Bladder Channels. It clears Heat and dissolves Toxins, benefits Water and promotes urination, relieves swelling, arrests seepage (i.e. stops bleeding, *Dai Xia*, and diarrhea), clears Heat and transforms Phlegm in the treatment of Lung Phlegm Heat, and relieves pain, inflammation, and swelling in traumatic injury. In this formula, Plantain aids Acacia in clearing Heat and eliminating Dampness from the Lower Burner/Large Intestine.

Herba Cardui Benedicti (Blessed Thistle) is Bitter, slightly Acrid, and Cool and enters the Liver/Gallbladder. It clears Heat and eliminates Dampness, especially from the Liver/Gallbladder. It benefits Water and promotes urination, relieves swelling and combats cancer. It promotes the eruption of pox and clears Heat from the *Shao Yang Fen*.

Flos Caryophylli (Cloves) is a TCM medicinal. It warms the Middle and descends Rebellion. In addition, it warms the Kidneys and aids the Yang. In this formula, Cloves prevent the Heat-clearing ingredients from harming the Righteous Fire of the Middle and Lower Burners. In addition, it assists in the production of Postnatal Kidney Yang, a process initiated in the Large Intestine.

Flos Trifolii (Red Clover) is Sweet, Bland, and Cool. It enters the Liver and Lungs. It clears Heat and dissolves Toxins, benefits Water and promotes urination, clears Heat from the Liver, disperses Accumulations, relieves swelling, and combats cancer. In addition, it benefits the throat and stops coughing due to Mutual Arising of Liver/Lung Heat. Red Clover stops *Dai Xia* and spermatorrhea due to Damp Heat discharging downward. It also relieves depression. In this formula, Red Clover assists Blessed Thistle in clearing Heat from the Liver, remembering that in young and middle-aged American adults, Liver Stagnation is the most common cause of constipation. Red Clover also assists Acacia and Plantain in eliminating Dampness from the Lower Burner.

Radix Rumicis (Yellow Dock) is also a Chinese herb but one only encountered in the *Kang Ai* or cancer-combatting pharmacopeia. It is Acrid, Bitter, and Cool. It clears Heat and dissolves Toxins, purges Fire and promotes bowel movements, disperses Stagnant Blood, relieves swelling, stops pain, stops itching, and kills Worms.

Cortex Juglandis Cinereae (Butternut Bark) is Bitter and Cold and enters the Stomach, Large Intestine, and Liver. It purges Fire and promotes bowel movements. It is useful for chronic constipation accompanied by Liver Congestion. Therefore, its functions are somewhat similar to Rhizoma Rhei.

This Western herbal formula is well crafted even for a TCM prescription. It addresses the main causes of Large Intestine dysfunction in young and middle-aged patients while at the same time being buffered so as to protect the Middle Burner. In addition, it also addresses the relationship between the Large Intestine and Kidney Yang and, therefore, the *Jing* Essence.

Yerba Prima's Colon Care Formula consists of three categories of ingredients: fiber or bulking agents, calcium, and intestinal bacteria. We have already discussed the use of intestinal bacteria above. In particular, Yerba Prima's Colon Care Formula consists of Lactobacillus Acidophilus, Lactobacillus Casei Var. Rhamnosis, Bifidobacterium Longum, and Enterococcus Faecium. Calcium Carbonate and Calcium Citrate are used to enable these bacteria to escape being destroyed by the stomach acid. The bulking agents (Psyllium Husks, Barley Fiber, Guar Gum, Oat Bran, and Fruit Pectin) all moisten the Intestines and promote bowel movements.

During the first week of this program, one takes 1 Kalenite tablet with 8 oz. of water BID between meals. Also 1 heaping teaspoon of Colon Care Formula is mixed in another 8 oz. of water and drunk immediately. (If not drunk immediately, it will stiffen up or set like jello.) This likewise should be taken between meals.

During weeks 2 & 3, one takes 2 Kalenite tablets 2-3 times per day and 1 heaping teaspoon of Colon Care also 2-3 times per day.

During weeks 4 to conclusion of the program, one takes 3 Kalenite tablets TID and 1 heaping teaspoon TID of Colon Care. This program should be followed for 2-3 months for best results. If, when beginning this program, there is intestinal gas, headaches, or worsening of any signs and symptoms, the patient should reduce the dosages of these medicinals and drink more water.

In addition to Kalenite tablets and Colon Care, I also typically recommend drinking Yerba Prima's Aloe Vera Juice Plus Herbs or Eagle Marketing's Oxy Toddy. Yerba Prima's Aloe Vera Juice Plus Herbs consists of Aloe Vera Juice, Peppermint, Parsley, and Chaparral.

Herba Aloes as used in TCM is the dried concentrate of Aloe Vera Juice. It purges Fire and moves the stool, clears Heat and cools the Liver. In Chinese medicine, it is classified as a strong cathartic and even a little of this concentrate can be quite purging. Aloe Vera Juice, however, because it is not a concentrate, is much milder although it has the same TCM functions. Aloe Vera is especially useful when constipation is due to Heat and Congestion of the Liver negatively influencing the Large Intestine as it so often is. Aloe Vera Juice has been used in the treatment of HIV. In one clinical trial, its use enabled 4/5 of its subjects to return to work.[1] It is not clear if this was due to Aloe Vera's having a direct anti-viral effect. My opinion is that Aloe Vera helps to regulate the Large Intestine and thus the *Zheng Qi* through the *Ming Men Zhi Huo*.

Folium Menthae Piperitae (Peppermint) is not identical to Herba Menthae in TCM. The latter is a species of Fieldmint or Horsement. However, these two related medicinals have essentially the same TCM functions except that Peppermint is better for relieving Constrained Liver Qi and harmonizing the Liver and Stomach.

Radix Petroselini (Parsley Root) is slightly Sweet and Warm. It enters the Liver, Gallbladder, and Stomach Channels. It regulates the Qi, dredges the Liver, and harmonizes the Stomach. In addition, it clears and eliminates Damp Heat from the Liver/Gallbladder and promotes urination, thus eliminating stones and relieving swelling.

Chaparral has already been discussed above under external applications for cervical dysplasia.

The addition of Aloe Vera Juice Plus Herbs to Yerba Prima's Internal Cleansing Program allows this program to deal more effectively with Liver Qi, Liver Heat, and Liver Depression. Since Liver Stagnation is such a common component of most modern patients' condition, I find this a necessary modification to the overall program and it takes into account the Liver and Large Intestine's mutually reflexive relationship.

Eagle Marketing's Oxy Toddy is another Aloe Vera Juice product I often recommend to patients undergoing colon cleansing. It is composed of Aloe Vera Juice, food grade Hydrogen Peroxide, and Pau D'Arco tea plus vitamins, minerals, and amino acids. We have already discussed the TCM functions of Pau D'Arco above under candidiasis. Hydrogen Peroxide, however, is a very interesting medicinal. Hydrogen Peroxide differs from water in that there are 2 oxygen atoms to this molecule (H_2O_2) instead of the one in plain water (H_2O). Hydrogen Peroxide is a very powerful anti-microbial agent when used both topically and internally. Most people have used it topically at least on inflamed wounds and skin infections. Many others use Hydrogen Peroxide along with Baking Soda to brush their teeth. Some alternative doctors both in Europe and the United States use Hydrogen Peroxide and/or Ozone (O_2) in the treatment of various cancers. Based on Hydrogen Peroxide's current medicinal uses and on my own personal experience, I think its TCM description is that it is Acrid, slightly Bitter, and Warm and that it kills *Chong* or parasites in their broad sense and that it dissolves Toxins.

Some practitioners may at first be perplexed at this description since most *Jie Du* or Toxin-dissolving medicinals in the Chinese *Ben Cao* are Cool or Cold. However, Warm Jie Du ingredients can be found under the expelling Worms (*Qu Chong*) category of medicinals in Chinese medicine. For instance, Bulbus Alli Sativi (Garlic) is Acrid and Warm and expels Worms and dissolves Toxins. This is an example of how some medicinals have a special empirical action which is otherwise not accounted for by the ingredients taste or temperature. In Ayurvedic medicine, such empirical efficacy which cannot be otherwise accounted for energetically is called a medicinal's *prabhava*. This concept of *prabhava* is an important one which might well be added to TCM since there are exceptions to the rule *vis a vis* certain medicinals' energetics in clinical practice. In any case, Hydrogen Peroxide is a potentially important medicinal which can be used for other than topical use. It is especially useful in dealing with parasitosis and yeast.

The above colon cleansing regime helps restore balance to the entire Triple Heater. It tonifies the Kidneys indirectly and strengthens the *Jing* Essence. It rids Evil Dampness and Heat and disperses Liver Excess. It facilitates ascension of the Pure and descension of the Turbid. In Western naturopathy, colon cleansing is one of the foundations of therapy. This approach to therapy has for too long been overlooked by TCM. Its inclusion in a TCM treatment plan extends the comprehensiveness and therapeutic efficacy of TCM.[2]

EXERCISE & DEEP RELAXATION

These two therapies should be continued essentially the same as during remedial therapy. They should be considered lifetime regimes. Basically, they are the regulation of rest and activity or Yin and Yang. When combined with proper diet, these three are the foremost factors in restoring and maintaining health.

Some readers may wonder where the patient's Spirit in a pyschospiritual sense comes into this regime. It is my belief based on experience that the Spirit is best served by promoting deep relaxation. When one is able to stay relaxed during thick and thin, the Qi flows unimpeded and regularly and everything goes where it should and does what it should. This is the deeper meaning of *Li Qi* or Qi regulation. The character *Li* means principle in the sense of innate, existentially mandated principle or natural law. When the Qi is *Li*, it flows according to its inherent *Dao* or Path. For this to happen, all any of us need to do is relax. Releasing held Qi, it will flow naturally within and according to its *Dao*. Thus all things under Heaven are accomplished *Wu Wei*, without doing.

HERBAL MEDICINE

For me, there are three basic issues to be addressed by internal herbal therapy in women who have recently gotten a good Pap after previously being diagnosed as having CIN. The first is continued rebalancing of their basic TCM *Zheng* or Pattern (of Disharmony). The second is the discriminating use of known anti-viral medicinals in an attempt to keep HPV and HSV II latent or inactive. And the third is occasional dispersion of Accumulation and Stagnation even if there are no obvious signs of such Accumulation and Stagnation.

1) Continued Rebalancing

Although Chinese medicine seeks to establish healthy balance within the organism, this balance is never achieved in any absolute way. We are constantly being influenced by a myriad of stimuli, each of which necessitates adjustment and rebalancing. In addition, we are each born with certain innate, constitutional imbalances. These are what make each of us different and create the dynamic of our lives. And, on top of constant conditional stimuli and innate constitutional factors, we here in the West are stressed beyond the natural carrying capacity of the human organism. Therefore, almost everyone can benefit from long-term herbal therapy.

In China, a person may get into a family fight, get upset, and come to the clinic with epigastric pain (*Wei Tong*), a *Qing* tongue, and a wiry pulse. Treatment is given, the patient feels much better, and the wiry pulse disappears. However, here in the West, at least 90% of my patients have a wiry pulse (among other complicating qualities), and this wiriness does not go away even after symptoms are rectified and relative health restored. It is my opinion that, as long as this wiry quality persists, some further therapy (not necessarily but possibly herbal) is indicated, since it is my belief that a wiry pulse is pathological. Although individual healthy pulses may vary in size, strength, and speed, a wiry pulse denotes blockage and constriction which simply are not healthy.

Continued TCM herbal therapy for preventive maintenance is based on diagnosis by *Bian Zheng*. An appropriate guiding formula is selected based on the patient's Root Pattern. As long as there are no Branch symptoms demanding remedial attention and, therefore, individualized modification of the guiding prescription, such long-term herbal therapy can usually and should be accomplished by pills, tablets, and desiccated extracts at lower doses than during the previous remedial therapy.

The majority of my cervical dysplasia patients suffer from some variation of Liver Qi/Liver Heat as their ongoing Pattern (of disharmony). Therefore, I most frequently tend to prescribe some version of either Xiao Yao San or Chai Hu Gui Zhi Tang.

Xiao Yao San

If there is Liver Qi Congestion with Spleen Qi Deficiency, some element of Dampness, and Blood Deficiency but *no* Transformative or Depressive Heat, I most often prescribe Xiao Yao Wan manufactured at the Lan Zhou Chinese Medicine Works in Gansu Province, PRC. This is just the simple, unmodified Xiao Yao formula, first recorded in the *Tai Ping Hui Min He Ji Chu Fang (Imperial Grace Formulary of the Tai Ping Era)* of the Song Dynasty, made into pills. These can be purchased from any Chinese apothecary in any Chinatown. They can also be ordered from Mayway Trading Co. of San Francisco. This formula is also available as a desiccated extract from Qualiherbs who refer to it as Bupleurum & Tang Kuei Formula.

In cases where there is Depressive or Transformative Heat on top of simple Liver Qi, Spleen Deficiency, and Blood Deficiency, then Dan Zhi Xiao Yao San is the professionally accurate prescription. This is available from K'an Herbs as Relaxed Wanderer. It is likewise available from Qualiherbs as a desiccated extract under the name Bupleurum & Peony Formula. As mentioned above, Dan Zhi Xiao Yao San includes Moutan and Gardenia in addition to the basic ingredients of plain Xiao Yao San. Relaxed Wanderer, formulated by Ted Kaptchuk, has not only these additions but also includes:

> Radix Ligustici Chuanxiong
> Rhizoma Gastrodia Elatae
> Rhizoma Cyperi Rotundae

Cyperus and Radix Ligustici Chuanxiong (aka Cnidium) promote the circulation of Qi and Blood respectively and, therefore, extend this formula's ability to disperse Insubstantial Stagnation. This is called activating the Qi and Blood to disperse Stagnation and is the mildest method of such dispersal, as opposed to dispersing Stagnation to activate the Qi and Blood or even cracking Stagnation. Gastrodia pacifies the Liver and extinguishes Wind and, therefore, helps to settle Internal agitation.

It is my opinion that Relaxed Wanderer should only be used when there is some lingering tendency to Stagnant Blood and Transformative or Depressive Heat. If neither of these are present, unmodified Xiao Yao San is preferable, especially for long-term administration. In Chinese medicine, if an ingredient is not called for based on the required therapeutic principles in turn derived from the individual diagnosis, that ingredient will cause imbalance. Some people think that because traditional Chinese medicinals are called herbs they are safe and non-iatrogenic. But this is not true. If the wrong herbs are given, not only will they not achieve their desired effect, they will cause an injurious or deleterious effect. This is quite important since, in my experience, it is usually necessary to have dispersed Stagnant Blood and cleared any Evil Heat before a good or negative Pap is obtained. Therefore, most often, unmodified Xiao Yao San is preferable for long-term, preventive maintenance. If Dan Zhi Xiao Yao San is still indicated by *Bian Zheng*, this suggests to me that the patient is still in the remedial phase of therapy.

Chai Hu Gui Zhi Tang

Chai Hu Gui Zhi Tang has been discussed above. In its original *Shang Han Lun* form, it is available as a desiccated extract from Qualiherbs under the name Bupleurum & Cinnamon Combination. It is also available as two slightly modified pills. Health Concerns markets its version as Ease 2 Bupleurum & Cinnamon Combination. Red Dates have been deleted from this version and Radix Puerariae added. The addition of Pueraria helps relieve shoulder/neck tension and also helps stop any tendency to loose stools.

Seven Forests of Portland, OR manufactures a pill they call Bupleurum 12 which is distributed by Health Concerns. It likewise omits the Red Dates and adds:

> Sclerotium Poriae Cocoris
> Rhizoma Atractylodis Macrocephalae
> Radix Angelicae Sinensis

Fructus Citri Seu Ponciri

Poria and Atractylodes aid Ginseng in tonifying the Spleen while at the same time eliminating Dampness through both transportation and transformation respectively. Dang Gui aids Peony in nourishing the Blood and relaxing the Liver. While Fructus Citri Seu Ponciri cracks Qi Stagnation, descends Rebellion, and promotes bowel movements, thus aiding Bupleurum's dredging and regulating the Qi. Although I might have preferred Dr. Dharmananda's not including Fructus Citri Seu Ponciri in this formula since, for long-term use, it may injure the Qi, still, I like this modification of Chai Hu Gui Zhi Tang especially for treating women with a chronic Liver/Spleen dyscrasia.

Heavenly Water

A major variation of Chai Hu Gui Zhi Tang is Heavenly Water or Gotu Kola 15 Formula created by myself and manufactured and marketed by Health Concerns. This formula is designed to address the same complicated disease mechanisms or *Bing Ji* as Chai Hu Gui Zhi Tang but includes ingredients more specific to the treatment of PMS and emotional stress. It avoids Bupleurum which can be too drying for women with borderline Blood and Yin Deficiency and intentionally enlists the Lungs' ability to control the Liver via the *Ke* cycle. Its ingredients are:

    Radix Hydrocotylis Asiaticae
    Herba Passiflorae Incarnatae
    Radix Pseudostellariae Heterophyllae
    Radix Scutellariae Baicalensis
    Rhizoma Pinelliae Ternatae
    Sclerotium Poriae Cocoris
    Radix Paeoniae Albae
    Radix Angelicae Sinensis

Rhizoma Cyperi Rotundi
Radix Trichosanthis Kirlowii
Fructus Zizyphi Jujubae
Radix Praeparatus Glycyrrhizae
Pericarpium Citri Reticulatae
Pericarpium Viridis Citri Reticulatae
Fructus Viticis Agnus-casti

Gotu Kola (Radix Hydrocotylis Asiaticae) is the ruler of this prescription. In many ways it is quite similar to Bupleurum. Both are Umbelliferates. Gotu Kola is likewise Cool and Acrid. Also like Bupleurum, Gotu Kola enters the Liver and Gallbladder Channels. It clears Heat, dissolves Toxins, stimulates the production of Body Fluids, and transforms Phlegm. However, it also relaxes constrained Liver Qi and relieves depression. It is especially useful for promoting mental calm and it relieves nervousness. Michael Tierra goes so far as to say that Gotu Kola possesses Yin tonic properties.[3] However, I would simply say it possesses all the Qi-regulating properties of Bupleurum without Bupleurum's drawbacks. In Indian Ayurvedic medicine, Gotu Kola is the most important nervine.

Passion Flower (Herba Passiflorae Incarnatae) is not a traditional Chinese herb but we can say that it is a *Li Qi* or Qi-regulating medicinal. It is Bitter and Cool and enters the Heart and Liver Channels. It extinguishes Wind and alleviates spasms, clears Heat and pacifies the Liver, and releases the Exterior. It treats depression, muscular tension, insomnia, restlessness, headache due to Hyperactive Yang, and is especially good for the long-term treatment of menstrual complaints, including PMS and dysmenorrhea.

Pseudostellaria (Radix Pseudostellariae Heterophyllae) is a *Bu Qi* or Qi-tonifying medicinal. It is Sweet and Neutral and enters the Spleen, Lung, and Heart. It strengthens the Spleen and benefits the Qi, while at the same time it generates Fluids. Shaolin Patriarch De Chan felt it was better to use Pseudostellaria rather than Ginseng or Codonopsis for women because it also cultivates the Blood.[4] Like American Ginseng, Pseudostellaria nourishes the Yin, but Pseudostellaria tonifies the Spleen more. Whereas, American Ginseng works primarily on the Lungs.

Scutellaria (Radix Scutellariae Baicalensis) is categorized as a medicinal which clears Heat and dries Dampness. It is Bitter and Cold and enters the Heart, Lungs, Gall Bladder, and Large Intestine. It clears Heat and quells Fire, especially in the Upper Burner. This Heat typically arises from the Liver and Stomach below. Most adults have some chronic Evil Heat trapped in their Lungs and as long as this Heat remains, Lung function is somewhat weakened. Therefore, the Lungs fail to control the Liver, on the one hand, and house the *Po* or animal vitality on the other. When the *Po* is weak, the *Hun* and *Shen* both also become *Bu An* or agitated and restless.[5] Therefore, clearing Heat from the Lungs and Heart is often one of the most effective ways of indirectly treating Liver Qi and Heat. Although not traditionally described as entering the Liver Channel, I think the fact that Scutellaria clears Damp Heat in the Middle and Lower Burners associated with such Liver diseases as Yang jaundice and *Re Lin* or Damp Heat Urinary Disturbance; because it clears Heat to *An Tai* or calm the fetus in the Uterus which is primarily controlled by the Liver; and also because it treats the *Shao Yang* phase of a *Shang Han*, strongly suggests that Scutellaria does, indeed, enter the *Jue Yin*.

Pinellia (Rhizoma Pinelliae Ternatae) is Acrid and Warm. It enters the Stomach and Spleen Channels. Pinellia dries Dampness, transforms Phlegm, and descends Rebellious Qi. It harmonizes the Stomach to reverse Upward Perversion and also dissipates Nodules and reduces distention. Pinellia is used in this formula to help regulate ascension and descension and eliminate Dampness, thus promoting harmonious Stomach/Spleen function. Although Pinellia is categorized as a Cold Phlegm transformer, it has definite Qi-regulating properties as well.

Poria (Sclerotium Poriae Cocoris) is Sweet, Bland, and Neutral. It enters the Heart, Spleen, and Lung Channels. It is a Dampness-seeping medicinal which promotes urination and leeches out Dampness. Therefore, it supports Pinellia by ridding Dampness by another avenue. It strengthens the Spleen and harmonizes the Middle. It transforms Phlegm, especially Phlegm which has been drafted up by Liver Qi to the Heart, Lungs, or chest (and therefore the breasts). Poria also calms the Spirit and quiets the Heart. In this formula it assists Orange Peel in eliminating Congested Fluids in the Middle which block ascension and descension.

Peony (Radix Paeoniae Albae) is a Blood-tonifying ingredient. It is Bitter, Sour, and Cool. It enters the Liver and Spleen. Peony nourishes the Blood and pacifies the Liver. Liver Qi Congestion can be dredged with Qi-regulating medicinals and relaxed from within by Blood-tonifying medicinals. Peony does the latter, and when combined with Qi-regulators, achieves a fuller, rounder, gentler effect. Peony also restrains Yang from floating upward and to the Surface and such flushing upward of Yang Qi accounts for a number of premenstrual symptoms, such as headache, insomnia, and breast distention.

Dang Gui (Radix Angelicae Sinensis) also tonifies the Blood. It is Sweet, Acrid, Bitter, and Warm and enters the Heart, Liver, and Spleen. It tonifies the Blood and regulates the menses, while it also invigorates and harmonizes the Blood. Dang Gui moistens the Intestines and promotes bowel movements which likewise tend to move the Qi down and decongest the Liver. Dang Gui is used to treat irregular menstruation and dysmenorrhea and works synergistically with Peony to relax the Liver by nourishing the Blood.

Cyperus (Rhizoma Cyperi Rotundi) regulates the Qi. It is Acrid, slightly Bitter, Sweet, and slightly Warm. It enters the Liver and Triple Heater Channels and it activates the Qi and resolves constrained Liver Qi. In this respect, it helps to harmonize the Liver and Spleen. It regulates menstruation and alleviates pain, such as dysmenorrhea. Cyperus unblocks Qi in the chest and the lower abdomen. When coupled with Dang Gui, it treats irregular menstruation and dysmenorrhea due to Stagnation of Qi and Blood. However, it will not tend to cause problems as Cnidium will in women without Blood Stagnation or menoxenia.

Trichosanthes (Radix Trichosanthis Kirlowii) is a Heat-clearing, Hot Phlegm-transforming ingredient according to most materia medica. However, its use is larger than that categorization would tend to infer. Early *Ben Cao*, such as the *Shen Nong Ben Cao Jing*, made no distinction between Pericarpium, Semen, Fructus, and Radix Trichosanthis medicinally. Radix Trichosanthis is Bitter, slightly Sweet, Sour, and Cool. It enters the Lungs and the Stomach. It clears Heat and generates Fluids. It also dissolves Toxins and expels pus. But it also broadens the chest by unbinding the Qi and moistens the Intestines and moves the stool. In terms of PMS, Trichosanthis helps treat the hunger, acne, thirst, constipation, and irritability which all occur as complex manifestations of Stomach/Lung/Liver Heat. Trichosanthes is the source for trichosanthin or Compound Q which is being used experimentally in the treatment of AIDS. Because Trichosanthes is the major ingredient in a TCM formula for the topical treatment of herpes simplex I[6] and because this formula is very effective, I believe that Trichosanthes does have an anti-viral effect.

Red Dates (Fructus Zizyphi Jujubae) are commonly added to complex prescriptions to moderate and harmonize any harsh effects or side-effects the other herbs might have, especially on the Stomach/Spleen. However, Red Dates are quite important in their own right. They are a *Bu Qi* or Qi-tonifying ingredient which are Sweet and Neutral and enter the Stomach, Spleen, and Heart. They tonify the Spleen and benefit the Stomach while calming the Heart Spirit. This is because they nourish the *Ying* or Nutritive Qi and the Blood and moisten Dryness, therefore nourishing Heart Blood. Symptomatically, they are used in the treatment of hysteria, restlessness, and anxiety due to Heart Blood/Spleen Qi Dual Deficiency.

Honey-baked Licorice (Radix Praeparatus Glycyrrhizae) is Sweet and Warm and enters all twelve Regular Channels and especially the Spleen and Lungs. It is a Qi-tonifying medicinal which tonifies the Spleen and benefits the Qi. It also moistens the Lungs, soothes spasms, and moderates and harmonizes the properties of the other herbs in this formula. Because it is used here in its honey-baked form, it helps generate Fluids in the Stomach and protects the Stomach from any tendency for Cool and Bitter herbs to harm the digestion. When combined with Peony, as it is in this prescription, it relieves abdominal pain, intestinal spasm, and spasms in the calves and other muscles.

Orange Peel (Pericarpium Citri Reticulatae) is from the Qi-regulating category of traditional Chinese medicinals. It is Acrid, Bitter, Warm, and Aromatic. It enters the Spleen, Stomach, and Lungs. It activates the Qi and strengthens the Spleen. It dries Dampness and transforms Phlegm. In terms of PMS, Orange Peel directs the Qi downward and facilitates ascension of the Pure and descension the Turbid. In this formula, it works synergistically with Pinellia and Poria to eliminate Spleen Dampness, and with Cyperus and Trichosanthes to unbind Chest Qi so as to reduce breast distention.

Green Orange Peel (Pericarpium Viridis Citri Reticulatae) is an unripe form of orange or tangerine peel. It is Bitter, Acrid, and slightly Warm. It enters the Liver and Gallbladder Channels. It expedites the free flow of Liver Qi, breaks up and reduces Qi Accumulations, and eliminates Dampness and transforms Phlegm. It is stronger than regular Orange Peel in its Qi-regulating function, more strongly removing Stagnation. When coupled with Cyperus, it treats pain in the flanks or breasts due to Liver Qi. When both Orange Peel and Green Orange Peel are combined, they reduce breast swelling and distention even more -- Orange Peel along the course of the *Yang Ming* and Green Orange Peel along the course of the *Shao Yang* and *Jue Yin*.

Chaste Tree Berries (Fructus Viticis Agnus-casti) are Sweet, Bitter, and Neutral and enter the Liver and Spleen. They are not a traditional Chinese medicinal but probably should be considered a Qi-regulating ingredient. They dredge the Qi, activate the Blood, and regulate the menses. Because they relieve pent-up Qi which can transform into Depressive Fire, they can restore normal sexual desire. A woman can be frigid due to *Ming Men* Fire being depressed inside. This is the same mechanism that gives rise to cold hands due to stress. Also a woman can be hyperactive sexually because of Depressive Liver Fire inflaming Stomach and Heart Fires giving rise to Flaring of the *Ming Men*. Chaste Tree Berries regulate towards normalcy both these tendencies. Therefore we can say that they regulate the *Ming Men* Fire and its relation to the other *Zang Fu*. In particular, Chaste Tree Berries relieve premenstrual tension and dysmenorrhea. David Hoffman, author of *The Holistic Herbal*, is also of the opinion that they help restore balance to a woman's internal environment after the use of oral contraceptives.

When taken as a whole, this formula is intended to dredge and relax congested Liver Qi, to relieve depression and lower

Rebellious Qi, to eliminate Dampness and transform Phlegm, to clear Heat from the Stomach and Liver, to generate Fluids and nourish the Blood, to activate the Qi and destagnate the Blood, and to harmonize the Liver and Spleen, the Spleen and Stomach, the Stomach and Intestines, and the Qi and Blood. It is indicated for the treatment of PMS due to Liver Qi, Spleen Deficiency and Dampness, Blood Deficiency, and Transformative Heat disturbing the *Shen* arising from the Liver and Stomach. In addition, this formula also treats irregular menstruation, delayed menstruation, painful menstruation, and fibrocystic disease when due to the above same constellation of disease mechanisms.

Bupleurum S

One final *He Fang* or Harmonizing formula I find useful for preventive maintenance in women with a past history of cervical dysplasia and the Liver Qi Pattern described above is Seven Forests' Bupleurum S. Its ingredients are:

  Cortex Magnoliae Officinalis
  Pericarpium Citri Reticulatae
  Rhizoma Pinelliae Ternatae
  Rhizoma Atractylodis Macrocephalae
  Rhizoma Atractylodis
  Radix Saussureae Seu Vladimiriae
  Rhizoma Recens Zingiberis
  Radix Glycyrrhizae
  Radix Bupleuri
  Fructus Germinatus Hordei

As a modification of both Ping Wei San (Calm the Stomach Powder) and Mu Xiang Shun Qi Wan (Saussurea Regulate the Qi Pills), Bupleurum S primarily is for the treatment of Liver Qi complicated by more pronounced Spleen Dampness.

Although it is "tight storage" of *Jing* Essence which ensures maintenance of a Hidden Evil in its latent state, I categorically do not recommend attempting to tonify the *Jing* through the use of Kidney/Liver and *Jing* tonics such as Placenta Hominis and Plastrum Testudinis unless the patient's TCM *Bian Zheng* diagnosis itself indicates this approach. It should be remembered that Postnatal *Jing* is manufactured during sleep from any excesses of Qi and Blood left over at the end of the day. Because the manufacture of abundant Qi and Blood is based on the ascension of the Pure and the descension of the Turbid, I recommend regulation of the Qi in general and of the Middle in particular as the best, long-term way of nourishing and supporting the *Jing*. Liver/Kidney and *Jing* tonics tend to be hard to digest and upset the Middle Burner and thus can cause the opposite of their intended effect. Outside most cancer clinics in China are vendors selling live turtles as *Yin Jing* tonics. But the professional doctors inside typically warn their patients not to eat too much of these since they can ruin their digestion.

Altogether other herbal formulas may be more appropriate than the ones mentioned above for long-term rebalancing and preventive maintainence. The important thing is the selection of a guiding prescription based on a professional discrimination of Patterns. Depending upon the season, the phase of the moon, the phase within the menstrual cycle, and even the weather, more than one prescription may need to be used in sequence or rotation. Also, as the woman's health and, therefore, balance improves, the prescription should be changed to keep current with her present *Zheng*. In addition, there should also be periodic breaks in herbal therapy to prevent any toxic buildup and to allow the patient's metabolism to reset itself.

2) Anti-viral Medicinals for Preventive Maintainence

I use Health Concerns' Power Mushrooms for long-term anti-viral prevention and maintainence. This formula is composed of five types of fungus or mushrooms. Its ingredients are:

>Fructificatio Ganodermae Lucidi
>Sclerotium Polypori Umbellati
>Sclerotium Poriae Cocoris
>Fructificatio Lentini
>Fructificatio Tremellae

In Chinese medicine, there are a number of formulas composed of ingredients which all belong to a single or similar taxonomic category, such as Wu Zi Wan (Five Fruits Pills) or Wu Pi San (Five Peels Powder). Power Mushrooms are one of these. In terms of treating a hidden virus, Ganoderma and Lentinus (aka Shiitake) are the two main ingredients. Both have demonstrated some anti-viral activity *in vitro*, especially Shiitake. Some researchers suggest that Lentinus has a stronger anti-viral activity and Ganoderma a stronger anti-bacterial activity. However, preparations of both are being used experimentally with HIV infected patients. Yet Power Mushrooms formula is more complex and more beneficial than simply that it seems to kill or neutralize viruses. When analyzed according to TCM theory, I think this formula reveals itself to be superior to other tablets composed of only Lentinus or Ganoderma.

Ganoderma is the famous Ling Zhi mushroom, considered a longevity medicinal by the Daoists. In TCM terms, it tonifies the Spleen Qi and Heart Blood and benefits the *Jing* Essence. It calms the Spirit and benefits Wisdom. In modern TCM, it is believed to also protect against the development of cancer.

Poria (aka Hoelen) benefits the Spleen, seeps Water, and also calms the Spirit. It likewise is considered a cancer preventive and promotes longevity. In addition, it strengthens the Spleen and transforms Phlegm. Both it and Ganoderma strengthen the Spleen and nourish the Heart and, therefore, their functions are very complementary.

Polyporus (aka Grifola) promotes urination and seeps Dampness. It is indicated in the treatment of both *Dai Xia* and *Zhuo Lin* or *Re Lin*, Turbid Urinary Disturbance and Hot Urinary Disturbance. When combined with Poria above, the two together more effectively seep Dampness. Since Dampness can generate Heat, by seeping Dampness, the Heat of Damp Heat can likewise be cleared even though Poria is Neutral and Polyporus is only slightly Cool.

Lentinus is not usually regarded as a professional medicinal in polypharmacy TCM. Rather it is regarded more as a food, although a very healthy food. Only lately has it been used in tablet form as a medicinal. Shiitake is Sweet and Neutral and enters the Liver and Stomach. It tonifies the Qi and Blood and benefits the Stomach. In Chinese *Xin Yi* or New Medicine (a combination of TCM and modern Western medicine), it is believed to lower blood pressure and reduce cholesterol as well as help prevent cancer. In terms of preventing cancer, I think this means it also has some *Jie Du* or Toxin-dissolving properties as well. Since folk recipes for Shiitake are used for measles and fish poisoning, I believe this *Jie Du* function is substantiated. In addition, eating Shiitake is recommended for dysuria and hematuria. This suggests Shiitake's ability to both seep Dampness and possibly clear Heat to stop bleeding. In particular, Shiitake is believed to specifically counteract stomach and cervical cancers.

Tremella (White Tree Ear) is Sweet and Neutral. It generates Fluids and moistens the Lungs. It is a Yin tonic. It is indicated for the treatment of Yin Deficiency insomnia, Lung disease, Liver disease, and poor appetite. Because it treats insomnia and poor appetite, I believe we can say it nourishes the Heart and Stomach as well as the Lungs. In *Xin Yi*, it is believed to reduce cholesterol in the prevention of heart attacks.

Taken as a whole, these five "mushrooms" treat both Righteous and Evil Yin of all Three Burners. Pei Zheng-xue, chief editor of the *Xue Zheng Lun Ping Shi (Commentary on The Treatise on Blood Disorders)*, says,

> Qi and Water have the same foundational basis. In treating the Qi, we treat the Water, and vice versa.[7]

And again,

> In summary, if one sees to the circulation of Water, then there will be Qi circulation, and if the Water is arrested, then the Qi will be arrested. Only those who understand this should speak regarding the regulation of Qi.[8]

Therefore, Power Mushrooms prevent Stagnation of Dampness and consequently Stagnation of Qi and Heat and transformation into Phlegm. Because the Qi flows unobstructedly, its growth flourishes, thus transforming Blood and Yin and nourishing the *Jing*. When Qi transports and transforms Water properly, the Lungs, Spleen, and Kidneys flourish and the Heart Spirit is secure. Thus Evil Qi is not allowed to flourish and Hidden Evils remain latent. The fact that some of its ingredients belong to the *Kang Ai* or cancer-combatting category of Chinese medicinals and that some of them have demonstrated anti-viral activity only makes this formula even more specifically appropriate for treating *Fu Wen Xie* of the viral, venereal variety.

3) Occasional Dispersion of Accumulation & Stagnation

Jia Kun recommends adults take Ping Xiao Dan once or twice per year as a cancer preventive. When used preventively, it is taken at a dose of 3 g BID or 1 1/2 g TID for 7 days. As we have seen above, Ping Xiao Dan is a strongly activating and dispersing formula. When taken once or twice a year, it prevents a build-up of Stagnant Qi and Blood, Dampness, Heat, and Phlegm. When taken by women, I suggest it should be taken before the period, not after. In terms of annual cycles, it should also be taken in the Spring and not in the Winter. Practitioners prescribing this formula should take care with the elderly, infirm, and Deficient in whose case it should not be used, its dosage reduced, or administered in tandem with *Fu Zheng* medicinals.

In Ayurvedic medicine, the traditional medicine of the Indian subcontinent, there is a concept called *Ama*. *Ama* means a plethoric, Evil Excess which accumulates in the body with age. In TCM terms, this describes the tendency of Stagnant Blood and Phlegm to accumulate in most people as they age due to the decline of Qi to *Yun* (transport) and *Hua* (transform) these substances. In Ayurvedic medicine, a course of therapy to discharge or disperse such *Ama* is usually administered before any attempt to tonify the organism. This concept of *Ama* and its dispersal and elimination is a useful concept to add to TCM, especially *vis a vis* preventive medicine. Zhang Zi-he, the founder of the famous School of Attack & Purgation of the Jin-Yuan Dynasties, understood this concept in therapeutics even if TCM does not have a single word for it in quite the same way Ayurveda does.

TOPICAL MEDICINE

Topical herbal medicine is not necessary after having obtained a negative Pap. However, women treated for CIN who are nervous about its recurrence may want to apply something to their cervix on an occasional basis in order to feel confident about their situation. In such cases, I recommend applying either Cod Liver Oil (i.e. Vitamins A & D), Liquid Folate, or Ultradophilus and Metagenics' Mycelized Children's Vitamins to the head of a tampon to be left over-night in the week after the cessation of the period. Although this is probably not necessary, it does provide some psychological comfort which, in and of itself, is a positive benefit.

ORTHOMOLECULAR THERAPY

Pizzorno & Murray recommend a woman's taking 2.5 mg of Folic Acid per day for 3 months to 1 year after obtaining a healthy Pap. In addition, I usually have my patients fill out a Metagenics' Health Appraisal Questionnaire and then prescribe the appropriate supplements based on that, my understanding of these supplements as TCM medicinals, and Vega biokinesiology. As stated above, I do believe our modern lifestyle and environmental stresses exceed the healthy carrying capacity of our human organism and that, faced with such unnatural stresses, orthomolecular supplementation is a useful and even necessary adjunct to modern health care. In particular, it is important to maintain adequate levels of B Vitamins, C, Beta-carotene, and A, E, and Zinc.

HOMEOPATHY AND HOMOTOXICOLOGY

Homeopathy was created by Samuel Hahnemann in the 18th Century. It is based on administering neutral tinctures and tablets which have been impregnated with the electromagnetic vibration of medicinal substances. If herbal and allopathic medicinals are primarily zenomolecular (meaning the use of molecules different from those constituting the body) and vitamins and minerals are orthomolecular (meaning the administration of the same molecules constituting the body), then homeopathy is ultramolecular (beyond molecules) in that no molecule of the medicinal substance originally used to make the homeopathic titration actually remains in the tincture or tablet.

Although the concept of ultramolecular medicine may seem to some somewhat tenuous, nevertheless, homeopathic medicine has been used very successfully throughout the world for 200 years. In the last several decades, European researchers have formulated a number of compound homeopathic remedies which are broad spectrum and can be prescribed based on sophisticated bioelectronic Vegatesting and Vega biokinesiology testing (VBK). Using potentitized resonance filters, practitioners can test for and diagnose the presence of hidden viruses in specific body tissues and can identify disease processes long before standard Western MDs and often TCM practitioners can.

Because of the very subtle nature of homeopathic medicines and because homeopathy has concerned itself for 200 hundred years with the systematic eradication of hidden toxins from the body, I believe homeopathy may be one of the best, most clinically effective, and most cost effective ways of negating or even cradicating hidden viruses from the body. Apex Energetics of Glendale, CA markets a compound homeopathic remedy called Post Virotox which is designed to eliminate chronic, hidden viruses from the body, such as CMV, EBV, HPV, etc. Using Vegatesting or Vega biokinesiology, patients can be tested both for the on-going presence of specific pathogenic viruses and the effectiveness of this and other, related homeopathic, orthomolecular, and zenomolecular remedies. In clinical practice, other Apex remedies are usually prescribed in tandem, such as Immunotox, Immunosode, Lymphotox, Spleen/Blood Activator, and/or Female Balance. If these remedies test positive for effectiveness and tolerance and the patient then takes them for some time, they can then be retested to see if the hidden viruses' pathogenic influence on the organism has, indeed, been neutralized.

In my practice, I typically first use Chinese herbs and orthomolecular therapy combined with acupuncture to treat the cervix remedially. I then continue using herbs and orthomoleculars to remedy any other presenting conditions, such as PMS, dysmenorrhea, early periods, acne, headaches, etc. When the patient is well balanced and essentially symptom-free from a TCM point of view, I then test for the presence of such key toxins as HSV and HPV and use homeopathic and homotoxicological remedies to neutralize any pathogenic effect from these. This use of AK or applied kinesiological diagnosis and homeopathic treatment extends the range and depth of therapy beyond that normally achievable through "straight" or conventional TCM.

Homotoxicology is the blending of modern Western pathophysiology and clinical diagnosis with homeopathic medicines. It differs from classical homeopathy in several ways. In classical homeopathy, high potency, single remedies are used based on constitutional conformation. Such constitutional conformation tends to emphasize a prescription hierarchy of spirit, mind, emotions, and finally physical signs and symptoms. Homotoxicology as originally developed by Dr. Hans-Heinrich Recekeweg is the use of polypharmacy or composite formulas at lower potencies. Most homotoxicological remedies are composed of several different ingredients at different potencies, but all usually quite low by classical standards. These ingredients can be homeopathic singles, nosodes, sarcodes or *suis* organ preparations, homeopathically adjusted allopathic medications, gemmotherapeutics, Schussler cell salts, Bach Flower remedies, lithotherapeutics, homeopathically adjusted orthomoleculars, and Krebs cycle catalysts.

These compound remedies are formulated based on Western pathophysiology as well as on clinical experience and specifically are designed to address Western and (in the case of some of Apex Energetics' products) Chinese disease categories and physical signs and symptoms. Some of the ingredients are titrated beyond Avagadro's Number and so are truly ultramolecular, but others are at extremely small but still molecular doses similar to the "doses" of hormones circulating in the body.[9] As David Riley, MD and homeopathic physician states, "Homotoxicology works by reactivating the defense system of the body ..."[10]

For a number of years I resisted combining homeopathy with TCM. TCM's basic theory of therapeutics is founded on the principle of heteropathy or that one uses an equal, opposite energy to neutralize a pathogenic energy. This, in turn, is founded on a several passages in the *Nei Jing* where it says to use Cold therapy to treat Hot diseases, reducing therapy to treat Excess diseases, moistening therapy to treat Dry diseases, and so on. Classical homeopathy's theory of therapy is based on the idea that like cures like (*Similia similibus currantur*). According to this approach, ultra small doses of a substance which ordinarily cause a set of signs and symptoms can stimulate the body's natural healing instincts to cure these very same signs and symptoms. As therapeutic theories, heteropathy and homeopathy appear diametrically and irreconcilably opposed.

However, more recently it seems that this theory of like cures like is only one theory behind the composition of homeopathic remedies. Nowadays, medicinals in homeopathic doses are prescribed to treat the same signs and symptoms as those same medicinals in zenomolecular or orthomolecular doses. The homeopathic indications for Greater Celandine (Chelidonum Majus), Fringe Tree (Chionathus Virginieus), and Thuja (Thuja Occidentalis) are essentially identical to their zenomolecular use. Therefore, it seems to me in modern homeopathy and homotoxicology the issue of homeopathy versus heteropathy has become moot.

It is true that when dealing with nosodes and homeopathic preparations of chemical toxins and pollutants, like cures like seems to be the rule. Nosodes are homeopathic preparations of microbial pathogens and diseased tissue. They stimulate the neutralization of these same pathogens and disease states. Likewise, homeopathic preparations of chemical and environmental pollutants are meant to discharge from or neutralize these same toxins in the human organism. The use of nosodes is essentially similar to the use of vaccinations. Vaccinations were used in China as early as the Tang Dynasty and again became popular in the 16th Century, one hundred years before they were introduced in the West.[11] This is at least one instance in Chinese medicine where like is used to cure like. Additionally, in Chinese medicine organ meats are used to tonify Deficiencies in their related Organs. Although this is based on adding something to fill a lack, it is not really heteropathy *per se* since the same substance is used to rectify the diseased Organ or Tissue. These contradictions in therapeutic principle in both Chinese and homeopathic medicines underscores the fact that there is more than one valid approach to therapeutics and that heteropathy and homeopathy are not, in the living organism, mutually exclusive or even accurately descriptive. Both have their use based on empirical results.

For me, the difference between zenomolecular therapy, as in Chinese and Western herbalism, and homeopathic therapy is merely one of dose. In Oriental medicine, we already have an emerging body of theory that suggests that the smaller the dose of a medicinal, the subtler and deeper the effect on the patient's organism. TCM uses large doses in polypharmacy formulas. *Kampo*, the Japanese version of Chinese herbal medicine which mostly uses *Jing Fang* or classical prescriptions from the *Shang Han Lun* and *Jin Gui Yao Lue*, uses one third or less the amounts that TCM practitioners do for the same formulas. This is based on contemporary TCM practitioners focusing on the speedy relief of major presenting complaints or *Biao* treatment and *Kampo* practitioners focusing more on asymptomatic *Ben* treatment. This idea has also been promoted by Ted Kaptchuk in the product guide to his Jade Pharmacy line of remedies. Dr. Kaptchuk says that the smaller the dose of a remedy the more subtle its influence on the organism. The schema Dr. Kaptchuk uses is that at smaller doses, medicinals effect less the gross physical body and more the mind, emotions, and eventually the Spirit.[12]

Homeopathic medicines are attenuated to much smaller doses than even Dr. Kaptchuk recommends and, therefore, I think do address more subtle layers of the human organism. Conventional TCM does not seem to have very good remedies for dealing with truly Hidden Evils other than to keep them latent. It is difficult to come up with a TCM treatment that specifically addresses such Hidden Evils while they are asymptomatic and attempts to eradicate them from the body. This inability is based on the limitations of the Four (Methods of) diagnosis and the modern rendering of *Fu Xie* as a "latent" Evil. Latent suggests that the pathogen is inactive. However, current research suggests that these viruses, although hidden, are not truly latent. Rather they are subtly and persistently damaging their host organism even though it may takes many years before this damage becomes obviously apparent to either Western or TCM clinicians. It is my hope and preliminary experience that homeopathics can reach and treat on subtler levels than conventional TCM therapy does. If this is true, then there is no reason why homeopathy cannot be combined with TCM. I believe the distinction between it and more standard TCM medicinals is only a matter of depths and dosages.

Apex Energetics runs training seminars in this method of diagnosis and therapy around the United States. More and more acupuncturists and TCM practitioners are adding homeopathy to their practice. In California, there is even a legislative push to include homeopathy in acupuncturists' legal scope of practice. On the other hand, some homeopaths believe that any zenomolecular and most orthomolecular therapy is detrimental to the immune system and that these therapies only suppress disease which then vicariate into other, deeper, more serious diseases. Although this may happen if zenomolecular or orthomolecular therapy is misapplied, it is my opinion that herbal and orthomolecular therapy administered based on a correct *Bian Zheng* diagnosis do not cause progressive (i.e. pathologic) vicariation. The problem is not with the herbs or orthomoleculars themselves, but with the correctness of their administration. In TCM, correct therapy can be proven through the Four (Methods of) diagnosis. If, after therapy, not only do the main presenting complaints abate, but all the other body functions, tongue, and pulse move towards healthy parameters, then this indicates reverse vicariation and not symptomatic suppression. Each group tends to focus inward and to develop an attitude that only they have the correct way. This is a dangerous attitude in any endeavor and particularly in health care. For a New Medicine for the 21st Century to arise, we must transcend these territorial limitations.

ACUPUNCTURE

Once a negative Pap smear has been obtained, I usually do not press the patient to continue acupuncture. That is not because I do not think acupuncture is effective therapy. It is. Rather, I am concerned with my patients' pocketbooks and worry about overburdening them with costly therapy. Instead, I try to emphasize the Three Free Therapies -- diet, exercise, and deep relaxation -- for long-term health maintainence and disease prevention.

However, should the patient want to continue with acupuncture, I typically focus specifically on *Jing Luo Zheng* or Channel & Collateral Patterns, Five Phase dyscrasias, and constitutional imbalances not particularly amenable to TCM herbal therapy. *Jing Luo* Pattern identification and treatment are not the forte of modern TCM acupuncture. By *Jing Luo Zheng*, I mean Patterns involving not just the *Shi Er Zheng Jing* (12 Regular Channels) but also the *Qi Jing Ba Mai* (Eight Extraordinary Vessels), the 15 or 16 *Luo Mai* (both Transverse and Longitudinal), the 12 *Jing Jin* (Channel Sinews), and the 12 *Jing Bie* or Channel Divergences. For a fuller discussion of this style of pre-TCM acupuncturist's acupuncture, the interested practitioner should see Mark Seem's *Acupuncture Imaging*.[13] For more information on Five Phase treatments, see Matsumoto and Birch's *Five Elements and Ten Stems*.[14] Constitutional acupuncture is discussed below under preventive therapy for men.

My and Dr. Seem's experience is that this kind of acupuncture frees up a person's Qi flow (and, therefore, mind/Spirit) in a way no other therapy does so directly and immediately. Such harmonization effects both the psyche and soma. Diagnosis in this type of pre-TCM acupuncture is largely based on palpation -- palpation of the body and the pulse-- and visual inspection of the patient's carriage and body symmetry. When doing this kind of acupuncture, it is best not to over-treat but rather to allow the patient time after a few treatments to further integrate the healing benefits catalyzed or set in motion by a few, skillfully selected points.

In addition, I often recommend patients to come in for "seasonal acupuncture tune-ups". At our clinic, we publish a newsletter at the turn of each Chinese season outlining the lifestyle guidelines given in the *Nei Jing* for the next 90 days.

Having patients come in every 90 days allows me to stay current with their situation, to record any changes in their tongue and pulse, and to give whatever encouragement is needed to keep the patient on their maintainence program. As long as the patient is asymptomatic, I mostly administer acupuncture tune-ups based on the pulse and *Hara*.

Addendum: During the preparation of *Sticking to the Point*, I came across an acupuncture combination given by Dr. Xi Yang-jiang of the Shanghai College of TCM during a lecture in San Francisco a number of years ago. This combination is Guan Chong (TH 1) and Shao Shang (Lu 11) for dispelling "Latent Toxins from the *Zang Fu*".[15] I have attempted to use this combination in asymptomatic HIV positives, HSV II infected persons during the hidden phase of that virus, and in women who have been diagnosed as having dysplasia, have been treated, and who are now ostensibly asymptomatic. When I have used these points together, it has been to dispel any lingering *Fu Wen Xie*.

My assumption regarding these points is that their use is meant to exteriorize these Inner Evils (*Nei Xie*) and bring them to the Surface where they can be neutralized or eliminated by the *Zheng Qi* and particularly the *Wei Qi*. This line of therapy is, I believe, what AZT and Compound Q do in HIV positives -- AZT with unacceptable benefit/risk ratio and Compound Q, for the most part, without injuring the *Sui* Marrow. Such exteriorization is routinely done in such viral, Hot, Toxic *Wen Bing* as measles and chicken pox where Surface-relieving medicinals are used to flush the pathogens to the Surface and then, in theory, from the body. This is called transmission from Inside to Outside in Chinese medicine. Medicinals which achieve such exteriorization are Acrid and dispersing. They catalyze the Lung Qi's clearing and dispersing function. Because of this, they tend to be drying and to injure the Qi, Blood, Fluids, and Yin.

During such exteriorization or reverse vicariation, skin rashes, muscle aches, fever, and other fluey feelings are the sign that the pathogens have been dispersed outwards to the Surface and that the *Wei Qi* is struggling with it. The following is my line of rationalization as to how these two points in tandem may achieve this effect.

Shao Shang is the Wood point on the Metal Meridian. This means it is capable of mobilizing Lung Qi to the Liver. This influx of Lung Qi across the *Ke* cycle causes the Liver Qi to disperse and with it the Blood. The Blood then moves towards the Surface, remembering that *Fu Wen Xie* reside in the *Xue Fen*. Secondly, dispersing Guan Chong, the Metal point on the Yang Fire Channel, mobilizes Qi to the Large Intestine. This influx of Fire Qi helps bolster the production of Kidney Yang and *Wei Qi* through the Internal Gate of the Triple Heater associated with the Large Intestine. This then causes exteriorization of the *Wei Qi* and Yang upward and outward similar to tonifying Fu Liu (Ki 7) to initiate sweating.

However, to date, this combination has not achieved such reverse vicariation in any of my HIV positives, HSV II positives, or HPV positives, at least not as evidenced by any of the above criteria. As of this writing, I am beginning to screen both HSV and HPV infected patients with biokinesiology using homeopathic nosodes of HSV II and HPV to see if those testing positive "go negative" after one or more treatments with these points. At the moment it is too early to tell if there is any effect of acupuncture utilizing this point combination on such lingering viruses.

MASSAGE

I am a great proponent of the healing benefits of regular massage. Quite frankly, I feel weekly massage is more therapeutically beneficial than weekly, repetitive TCM acupuncture. Massage regulates the flow of Qi, Blood, and Liquids at the same time as it calms the *Shen* and relaxes the *Jin* and, therefore, the Liver. It also benefits the digestion and promotes bowel movements. In addition, massage nourishes a person emotionally in a way no other therapy can. As healers, we must never underestimate the value of nurturing, caring touch and the shared human solidarity it conveys.

For emotionally stressed patients with tight muscles and wandering, chronic aches and pains, I recommend oil massage. These patients generally suffer from an Excess accumulation of Qi and its subsequent erratic or rebellious flow. Such patients tend to be more Yang and less Yin. Oil massage smoothes and regulates the flow of Qi as well as nourishes substance or Yin. However, for obese patients, oil massage is contraindicated since, because it increases substance, it can also increase Phlegm and Dampness. In such cases, Shiatsu is definitely beneficial to stimulate and invigorate the flow of Qi. Obese patients are more Yin and less Yang. They need to be energized and circulated rather than smoothed and dampened. This opinion about these two types of massage is based on a Yin Yang understanding of them *vis a vis* energy and substance and on Tibetan medical theory concerning massage.

SEX

Oriental medicine, whether Chinese, Tibetan, or Ayurvedic, counsels against sex during menstruation. During menstruation, the flow of Qi and Blood in the *Chong* and *Ren* is downward. Sex typically reverses this flow. This then results in Qi and Blood Stagnation. Since Qi and Blood Stagnation so often complicates the TCM Patterns which present with cervical dysplasia, it seems wise to avoid anything which might cause or exacerbate them. Although some Westerners may question the validity of this theory, deeming it a cultural or sexual bias, my patient histories over the past 10 years tend to confirm that, as Oriental medical theory holds, sex during menstruation is linked with increased incidence of Uterine Qi and Blood Stagnation.

In addition, since cervical dysplasia seems to be, at the very least, in part a venereal disease, it is my advice to my dysplasia patients that they not have sex with multiple or casual partners without the use of condoms. As mentioned above, even women in monogamous relationships who have had positive Pap smears should consider the use of condoms until their male sexual partners have been checked and treated for HPV infection. Unfortunately, subclinical males may be resistant to such diagnosis and treatment if they have no obviously visible lesions.

REPEAT PAP SMEARS

Women who have had a bad or positive Pap smear and who have undergone successful remedial therapy for CIN should get 2 repeat Pap smears at 3 month intervals. After that, they should receive a third Pap 6 months later before resuming a regular once a year bimanual exam *cum* Pap smear.

Officials from the Colorado State Department of Health working in epidemiology and cancer control have stated to me that no one should or needs to die from cervical cancer. If a woman dies from cervical cancer, it is due to a "system breakdown" which one staffer described as being a failure in either initial screening or loss to follow-up. Certain racial, cultural, and socio-economic subgroups do not get regular Pap smears as they should. Early detection of dysplasia is the key to successful treatment whether by modern Western medicine or Traditional Chinese Medicine. The prognosis is largely dependent upon the depth of invasion of dysplastic cells and Pap smears are the best available, early screening test for such dysplastic cells. In addition, I think it quite likely that in the future most young adult women will be regularly screened by the ViraPap or some other such HPV DNA identifying test. I have also been told that there are several attempts at developing a serological test (blood test) for HPV infection but that such a test will probably not be available for several more years. Those testing positive for strains of HPV known to cause life-threatening malignancies should be followed all the more closely.

Loss to follow-up refers to women who have received a bad or positive Pap and then do nothing about it. Such lack of follow-up is usually due to lack of information or lack of understanding about the relationship of cervical dysplasia to cervical/uterine cancer and/or lack of money to pay for therapy. Although I believe Traditional Chinese Medicine treats cervical dysplasia more comprehensively than modern Western medicine, all women should get regularly scheduled Pap smears and should seek active treatment for any and all dysplasias no matter which medicine they choose to be treated by. Before the advent of the Papanicolaou test, cervical cancer killed more American women than any other cancer. Since the introduction of regular Pap smear screening, cervical cancer mortality has fallen to the bottom of the list. The Papanicolaou test is one Western medical diagnostic procedure I strongly recommend to all my female patients. Unfortunately, less than 40% of American women get yearly Pap smears.[16]

THE SILVER LINING

The good news is that women who are successfully treated for CIN may be immune to its recurrence. Persons with common skin warts which suddenly disappear are immune to their recurrence due to the development of sufficient antibodies. Such lifetime immunity is common with other viral diseases which have been successfully dealt with by the host organism, such as rubella, rubeola, and varicella. It is possible that this is also the case with anogenital strains of HPV.

If natural treatments, such as herbs, acupuncture, micronutrients, and homeopathics, result in a reversal of dysplasia and condylomata, this is due, in all probability to these therapies' immune-modulating effect and enhanced immune competence. Although chemodestructive and surgical destructive therapies may also provoke such a positive immune response, in a certain percentage of patients they do not. Therefore, for this reason as well, more natural, immune-modulating therapies may be superior.

Whether anogenital strains of HPV are similar in this regard to rubeola and varicella or to HSV I and II which only remit and can be reactivated has yet to be determined. I personally hope and pray that successful natural treatment does confer a lifetime immunity to reinfection and recurrence. However, even if it does not, the preventive regimes discussed above should be able to maintain HPV in its latent state well into old age.

CHAPTER SIX
THE TCM DIAGNOSIS & TREATMENT OF GENITAL WARTS

This book has, so far, primarily focused on the treatment of cervical dysplasia. It has assumed that most, if not all, cervical dysplasia is due at least in part to HPV or some combination of HPV and other venereally transmitted pathogens in relation to a defect or compromise in the patient's immune response. However, many men and women suffer from the embarrassment, disfigurement, and discomfort of genital warts. Therefore, some discussion of the TCM diagnosis and treatment of obvious genital warts is in order.

DIAGNOSIS

As of this writing, I have not been able to find any specific discussion of genital warts in the TCM *Wai Ke* or *Pi Fu Ke* literature. *A Handbook of Traditional Chinese Dermatology* by Liang Jian-hui, under dermatoses due to viral infection, lists common warts, flat warts, infectious soft warts, filiform warts, and plantar warts, but not genital warts.[1] Reading the descriptions of these, there is no mention under any of these categories of genital occurrence. The TCM literature of which I am aware seems to be somewhat reticent on this issue.

Warts in general are called *Qian Ri Chuang*, Thousand Day Lesions in Chinese, since they sometimes disappear spontaneously after a protracted period of time. They are also called *Ci Hou* or Thorny Condition in the classics. This refers to the acanthosis typical of verrucae. All the above Chinese-identified species of warts have Wind as part of their etiology. In this case, Wind refers to an unseen pathogen and most definitely does not imply injury by physical or meteorological wind. In this sense, Wind Evil or *Feng Xie* is merely synonymous with *Xie Qi*. It should be remembered that the Chinese character for Qi is composed of a pictograph showing blowing wind.

Dr. Liang gives the *Bing Yin/Bing Ji* for common warts as lingering Wind Evil in the skin due to Blood Dryness and Liver Deficiency. This description is derived both from the physical appearance of common warts and the fact that they typically occur on the hands and feet and especially around the borders of the nails. The nails are the effluvia of the *Jin* Sinews which are most obvious and prominent in the hands and feet. The *Jing Jin*, it should be remembered, connect with the *Zheng Jing* or Regular Channels at the *Jing* Well points. The *Jin* are nourished by Blood and are the tissue related to the Liver. Genital warts arise on and around the genitals and anus. This area is irrigated by the Liver Channel itself and its Longitudinal *Luo*. Moreover, in men the penis is described as the union of the hundred *Jin*. There is a Pattern of impotence in Chinese medicine due to Malnourishment of the *Jin* causing inability of the penis to achieve erection. In addition, Dr. Liang says that flat warts or *Bian Hou* are caused by Wind Heat Toxins externally and Flaring Liver Fire internally.

Using a combination of both these *Bing Yin/Bing Ji*, I think we can develop a description of the TCM etiology and *Bian Zheng* diagnosis of genital warts. Besides involving a sexually transmitted *Fu Wen Xie* or *Li Qi*, I believe that genital warts can run the gamut from Liver Blood Deficiency plus Toxins to Liver Fire and Damp Heat plus Toxins. If the warts are pale and horny, slow growing, few and well-contained, they involve more prominent Liver Deficiency. On the other hand, if they are fast growing, proliferative, red, and inflamed, they are likely associated with Liver Fire. Whereas, if they are ulcerated, weeping, and wet as well as being red and inflamed, they are more likely associated with Damp Heat.

TREATMENT

Internal Herbal Medicines

Based on the above suggested *Bian Zheng* discrimination, systemic balancing and, therefore, immune-modulating therapy can be given using Chinese herbs and orthomolecular remedies internally. If the lesions themselves and the patient's tongue, pulse, and other, corroborating signs and symptoms suggest Liver Blood Deficiency, medicinals which tonify Liver Blood are indicated. If the tongue, pulse, signs and symptoms, and the lesions themselves suggest Liver Fire, medicinals which clear Heat from the Liver should be used. And, if the tongue, pulse, signs, symptoms, and lesions themselves suggest Damp Heat, medicinals which clear Heat and eliminate Dampness specifically from the skin and the Lower Burner should be chosen.

There are several Chinese herbal formulas I have found useful when administered internally for the treatment of anogenital warts. Many of these contain Coix or Job's Tears (Semen Coicis Lachryma-jobi, a species of Oriental barley). Coix is used empirically in Chinese medicine to both eliminate warts or verrucae and also to prevent and combat against cancer. The TCM description of Coix is that it is Sweet, Bland, and Cool and that it enters the Lungs, Spleen, and Kidneys. It promotes urination and leeches out Dampness, strengthens the Spleen and stops diarrhea, clears Heat and expels pus, expels Wind Dampness, and clears and eliminates Damp Heat.

Yi Yi Ren Tang (Coix Decoction, aka Coix Combination)

This formula is available from Qualiherbs as a desiccated extract. It is listed in Hsu and Hsu[2] and should not be confused with the formula of the same Chinese name listed in Bensky and Barolet.[3] This formula is most often prescribed for rheumatic complaints. However, it can also be used for warts, in which case it should be used at low *Kampo* or Japanese dosages. The ingredients in this formula are:

    Herba Ephedrae
    Rhizoma Atractylodis
    Radix Angelicae Sinensis
    Radix Paeoniae Albae
    Semen Coicis Lachryma-jobi
    Ramulus Cinnamomi
    Radix Glycyrrhizae

This formula achieves its effects by three lines of action. First, Ephedra disperses Lung Qi to the Surface, thus exteriorizing pathogens and transmitting them from Inside to Outside. At the Surface, these Evil Qi are neutralized by the *Wei Qi* activated by Ramulus Cinnamomi. Secondly, Dang Gui and Peony nourish the Blood and thus the skin. And third, Atractylodes and Coix eliminate Dampness, thus benefitting the Qi. Physically, warts are an accumulation of Yin which the Qi at the Surface is not sufficiently transporting and transforming. This formula energizes the Lung Qi's ability to permeate and transform this Yin Accumulation. In addition, we can also say that Coix does have an empirical anti-wart effect and that Licorice has an empirical and theoretical anti-viral, anti-Toxin effect.[4] This formula can be used in patients with Liver Excess insulting the Lungs with Spleen Dampness. It is indicated especially if the patient simultaneously complains of rheumatic problems and muscular spasms.

Ma Huang Yi Gan Tang   (Ephedra, Coix, & Licorice Decoction, aka Ma Huang & Coix Combination)

This formula is somewhat similar to the above. Its ingredients are:

    Herba Ephedrae
    Semen Pruni Armeniacae
    Semen Coicis Lachryma-jobi
    Radix Glycyrrhizae

Hsu and Hsu indicate this formula for the treatment of warts.[5] It works similar to Yi Yi Ren Tang by exteriorizing Evil Qi by catalyzing the Lungs' dispersion of the Surface. The difference is that it does not nourish the Blood but rather transforms Phlegm and moistens the Intestines, thus promoting bowel movements. This formula should likewise be administered at *Kampo* or Japanese dosages for the treatment of warts over a protracted period. It is especially indicated if the patient suffers concomitantly from rheumatism, neuralgia, dry skin, corns, and calluses, dandruff, and chronic respiratory complaints such as asthma with tenacious Phlegm.

Yi Yi Fu Zi Bai Jiang San   (Coix, Aconite, & Patrinia Powder, aka Coix, Aconite & Thlaspi Combination)

This formula is found under the *Yong Yang* or carbuncle/dermatosis category of Chinese formulas. In TCM, it is primarily used to treat Intestinal Abscess for which it is prescribed in large dosages. However, I find this a very important and useful formula for the treatment of *Shao Fu Tong* or Lower Abdominal Pain due to Mutual Entanglement of Dampness and Heat with Qi and Blood Stagnation in the Lower Burner. Hsu and Hsu list this formula for the treatment of leukorrhea, fungal diseases, and verrucae or warts as well as for Intestinal Abscess.[6] When it is used to treat anogenital warts, it should be prescribed at *Kampo* dosages. The ingredients in this formula are:

> Semen Coicis Lachryma-jobi
> Herba Patriniae Heterophyllae
> Radix Praeparatus Aconiti Carmichaeli

As mentioned above, Coix is a specific anti-wart medicinal in Chinese medicine. In addition, it eliminates Dampness and benefits the skin. Patrinia (aka Herba Baijiangcao, aka Thlaspi) is an anti-cancer medicinal which specifically addresses Mutual Entanglement of Dampness and Heat with Qi and Blood Stagnation in the Lower Burner. This is a very commonly encountered Pattern amongst American patients. Aconite, used here in very small amount, warms Kidney Yang. In this formula, it supports the Righteous warmth of the *Ming Men Zhi Huo* while Patrinia clears Heat from the Lower Burner.

The fact that this formula is primarily used to treat Intestinal Abscess in TCM once again underscores the close relationship of Kidney Yang to the Large Intestine and to the urogenital and reproductive tract as well. When used to treat *Shao Fu Tong* and *Tong Jing*, this formula can be modified by adding other Qi and Blood activating medicinals. However, when treating anogenital warts in patients without other prominent signs and symptoms, it can and should be administered as a desiccated extract in low but continuous doses. I find Patrinia a very important ingredient. In this formula it addresses the major Pattern, while Coix is specifically anti-verrucal.

Ban Xia Xie Xin Tang Jia Yi Yi Ren
 (Pinellia Disperse the Heart
 Decoction with Coix, aka Pinellia

Combination with Coix)

This formula is given by Keisetsu Otsuka *et al.* in *Natural Healing With Chinese Herbs* for the treatment of warts.[7] It is the very first formula I ever used for the treatment of anal warts when I first was in practice. At the time, I prescribed it based on the patient's over-all TCM diagnosis and complicating complaints -- gastritis and borborygmus. I was actually surprised when the patient reported several months later that not only had this formula benefitted his digestion but that his anal warts had disappeared. This formula is one of the basic 3 *Xie Xin* or Heart-dispersing formulas I use in correlation with Dr. Yoo's constitutional diagnosis. In the case of anal warts, this formula eliminates Damp Heat from the Large Intestine while the addition of Coix is specifically anti-verrucal. The ingredients in this formula are:

> Rhizoma Pinelliae Ternatae
> Radix Panacis Ginseng
> Radix Scutellariae Baicalensis
> Rhizoma Coptidis
> Radix Glycyrrhizae
> Fructus Zizyphi Jujubae
> Rhizoma Zingiberis
> Semen Coicis Lacryma-jobi

Teng Long Tang   **(Soaring Dragon Decoction, aka Moutan & Persica Combination)**

Soaring Dragon Decoction is also a *Yong Yang* formula and it too contains Coix. Hsu and Hsu indicate this prescription for the treatment of prostatitis and the initial stages of uterine cancer,[8] remembering that in Chinese medical texts no distinction is made between uterine and cervical cancers. It is also indicated for the treatment of periproctitis, testitis, peritonitis, endometritis, and uterine tumors. All these indications suggest an accumulation of Dampness, Heat, and Stagnant Blood in the Lower Burner. Soaring Dragon Decoction's ingredients are:

>   Cortex Radicis Moutan
>   Rhizoma Atractylodis
>   Semen Pruni Persicae
>   Semen Coicis Lachryma-jobi
>   Semen Benincasae Hispidae
>   Rhizoma Rhei
>   Mirabilitum
>   Radix Glycyrrhizae

This formula is likewise available from Qualiherbs as a desiccated extract. Because it contains Rhubarb and Mirabilitum, it should be used only in those with accompanying constipation.

Xiang Chuan Jie Du Ji   **(Fragrant River Toxin Dissolving Formula, aka Smilax & Akebia Combination)**

Xiang Chuan Jie Du Ji is a Japanese formula primarily for venereal diseases. Hsu and Hsu list its indications as syphilitic bubo, any syphilitic skin lesion, syphilitic keratitis, and gonorrhea.[9] Syphilitic keratitis or a horny cornification due to an STD suggests to me that this formula may be useful in treating venereal warts. Its ingredients are:

>   Rhizoma Smilacis Glabrae
>   Caulis Akebiae Mutong
>   Radix Ligustici Chuanxiong
>   Sclerotium Poriae Cocoris
>   Flos Lonicerae
>   Rhizoma Rhei

Radix Glycyrrhizae

This formula is for the treatment of sexually-transmitted Evil Qi and Damp Heat and Stagnant Blood in the Lower Burner. It once again takes into account the Large Intestine's crucial role in regulating the internal environment of all the pelvic contents.

Zi Gen Mu Li Tang (Lithospermum & Oyster Shell Decoction)

This is another Japanese formula. It treats syphilitic skin lesions or skin lesions due to STD and malignant skin diseases. In addition, it also treats lymphadenitis. Hsu and Hsu mention lymphadenitis in the neck. However, their diagram also shows lymph node enlargement in the groin as well.[10] Many persons with latent, sexually-transmitted *Fu Wen Xie* have chronically enlarged, nodular lymph nodes in their groin and this is how I discriminate the selection of this formula for the treatment of anogenital warts. The ingredients in Zi Gen Mu Li Tang are:

> Radix Angelicae Sinensis
> Radix Paeoniae Albae
> Radix Ligustici Chuanxiong
> Concha Ostreae
> Radix Astragali Seu Hedysari
> Radix Lithospermi Seu Arnebiae
> Flos Lonicerae
> Rhizoma Cimicifugae
> Rhizoma Rhei
> Radix Glycyrrhizae

Wen Jing Yin (Warm the Essence Drink, aka Tang Kuei & Gardenia Combination)

Wen Jing Tang is a commonly prescribed formula for the treatment of chronic skin conditions due to Blood Deficiency and lingering Dampness and Heat. Its ingredients tonify the Blood, nourish and relax the Liver, and benefit the Essence while at the same time clearing Heat from the Liver, Lungs, Stomach, and Heart. It is available from Qualiherbs as a desiccated extract. When treating anogenital warts, Coix can be added to make this formula more specific for that condition. Licorice and Astragalus can also be added to tonify the *Zheng Qi* and especially the *Wei Qi* and further dissolve Toxins in the skin. Wen Jing Tang's standard ingredients are:

>   Radix Angelicae Sinensis
>   Radix Paeoniae Albae
>   Radix Rehmanniae
>   Radix Ligustici Chuanxiong
>   Rhizoma Coptidis
>   Radix Scutellariae Baicalensis
>   Fructus Gardeniae
>   Cortex Phellodendri

Xiao Feng San   (Scatter Wind Powder, aka Tang Kuei & Arctium Formula)

This formula is usually prescribed for chronic Damp Heat skin lesions complicated by Blood Deficiency. However, Hsu and Van Benschoten indicate it for the treatment of "Hidden Blood rash"[11] which I read as a rash or skin lesion due to a Hidden Evil in the *Xue Fen*. This formula not only clears and eliminates Damp Heat but also exteriorizes or transmits Evil Qi from the Inside to the Outside. This is accomplished through the use of Arctium, Schizonepeta, and Cicada, all of which promote the exteriorization of skin "rashes" due to viral infection arising as Heat and Dampness from the Inside. The ingredients in this formula are:

Radix Angelicae Sinensis
Radix Rehmanniae
Rhizoma Anemarrhenae
Rhizoma Atractylodis
Fructus Arctii
Semen Sesami Indici
Caulis Akebiae Mutong
Radix Sophorae Flavescentis
Periostracum Cicadae
Flos Schizonepetae
Radix Ledebouriellae Sesloidis
Gypsum
Radix Glycyrrhizae

There are also two simple, single ingredient, anti-wart formulas I have recently common across which can be used in conjunction with the above treatments for anogenital warts. They fall somewhere between dietary and herbal therapy. The first is given by Henry C. Lu as an internal folk remedy for warts. Dr. Lu says to decoct 40 g of Coix in water, divide the resulting liquid into 2 doses, and take 1 dose BID for 10 days. A variation of this is to eat 60 g of Coix cooked with white rice once per day until recovery.[12]

The second prescription is given by Albert Y. Leung. Dr. Leung reports that patients with common warts in southeastern China were fed only plain, water-boiled yellow bean sprouts without salt or other seasoning TID for 3 days. On the fourth day, these patients were allowed to resume their normal diet. All the patients in this study subsequently recovered from their warts which did not reappear.[13]

External or Topical Treatments

When it comes to topical treatment of warts themselves,

Chinese medicine essentially uses the same treatment strategies as modern Western medicine: cauterization and escarosis. Direct moxibustion is used to burn off common warts and medicinals such as Fructus Bruceae Javanicae which are caustic and exfoliative are applied topically. Since laser vaporization, BCA therapy, and surgical excision are essentially identical in approach to these Chinese therapies, and, since these Western therapies are less painful and more efficient, I typically recommend patients to receive these Western therapies for the physical removal of genital warts.

For those patients and practitioners who prefer to first try TCM or naturopathic remedies, there are several topical treatments for warts which can be tried for anogenital warts. There are several herbal oils which can be applied once per day directly to the warts. These include Brucea Oil made by smashing Fructus Bruceae Javanicae and obtaining the oil, Tea Tree Oil, and Thuja Oil. All of these have demonstrated anti-wart activity. Or, tinctures can be made from Chaparral, Greater Celandine (Radix Chelidonii Majus), or Rhizoma Drynariae, aka Rhizoma Gusuibu. Bensky and Gamble mention the use of this last tincture in the treatment of warts and I have found it effective in some patients.[14] These tinctures are usually applied once or several times per day.

For those with both Blood Deficiency and Heat, unmodified Zi Cao Gao (Lithospermum Ointment) sometimes helps regress anogenital warts. Its ingredients are:

>Radix Lithospermi Seu Arnebiae
>Radix Angelicae Sinensis
>Lard
>Beeswax
>Sesame Oil

Lithospermum clears Heat and dissolves Fire Toxins. It also

clears and eliminates Damp Heat in the skin and cools the Blood, remembering that HPV as a *Wen Re Xie* resides in the *Xue Fen* or Blood Phase. Dang Gui nourishes and activates the Blood. While Lard, Beeswax, and Sesame Oil nourish and mollify the skin.

Fu Fang Zi Cao Gao or Modified Lithospermum Ointment is a formula with which I have been experimenting. It contains the same ingredients as regular Zi Cao Gao but also others which are meant to disperse Stagnation and Accumulation, dissolve Toxins, expel Wind, and generate New Tissue. Its ingredients are:

    Radix Lithospermi Seu Arnebiae
    Radix Angelicae Sinensis
    Radix Glycyrrhizae
    Radix Symphyti Officinalis
    Fructus Bruceae Javanicae
    Nidus Vespae
    Myrrha
    Gummum Benzoin
    Lard
    Beeswax
    Sesame Oil

In this formula, Brucea is an empirical specific for warts. It works by escarosis. Licorice is added both for its dissolution of Toxins in the skin and for its lenifying effect. Nidus Vespae dissolves Toxins and expels Wind. It enters the Liver Channel. Myrrh activates the Blood and disperses Stagnant Blood. When applied topically, it also promotes the generation of New Flesh. Comfrey Root also promotes the generation of New Flesh and thus helps to mitigate the caustic effects of Brucea, especially on surrounding healthy skin. Benzoin is used to penetrate Turbidity. Turbidity is a plethora of Yin. Warts are also a plethora of Yin. Benzoin helps to activate the Yang to transport and transform this Yin Accumulation. I and a number of other practitioners have had some success in using this ointment on warts, including anogenital warts.

When choosing surgery, a judgement must be made. Is the patient strong enough that such surgical trauma in fact stimulates their local cellular and systemic humoral immune response, thus not only removing the gross lesions but also stimulating regression of subclinical lesions? Or, is the patient's immune system already compromised to the point where the stress of surgical trauma weakens the immune response even more? Western doctors, it seems, make this determination by giving the escarotic or caustic therapy and seeing if new lesions appear week by week. Although this is one obvious, empirical method, tongue and pulse diagnosis might be able to determine this before weakening the immune system even further. Most wart patients are a mixture of Excess and Deficiency. The more Excess a patient is, the more likely it is that trauma will stimulate their *Zheng Qi*. The more Deficient a patient is, the more likely it is that trauma will cause even further insult and weakening. Deficient patients with a compromised immune system should be treated primarily with internally administered medicines coupled with, perhaps, Interferon injections or local vitamin injection (A or Folic Acid).

A final possibility for the treatment of anogenital warts is the local, subcutaneous injection of homeopathically prepared HPV nosode. Such injections can be given once per week similar to Interferon injections. Their intention is to stimulate the patient's own immune system to regress the condylomatous lesions.

After visible, clinical or subclinical lesions have been eliminated, Chinese herbal medicine, orthomoleculars, and homeopathic remedies may all be used to maintain immune-activated latency of any remaining HPV. Such therapy should be based on an individualized *Bian Zheng* diagnosis. since the immune system is none other than the *Zheng Qi* and the *Zheng Qi* is essentially synonymous with the *Yuan* Original Qi. Constitutional balancing ensures normal production of this *Zheng Qi* through ascension of the Pure and descension of the Turbid.

CHAPTER SEVEN
PROSTATITIS, PROSTATIC HYPERTROPHY, AND PROSTATE CANCER

If cervical dysplasia is a *Fu Xie Wen Bing* spread by sex, men must be equally infected. However, there is no male equivalent to the Pap smear to screen for and detect the early effects of such a Hidden Evil, at least not in the tissue for which I fear most -- the prostate. Rectal digital examination of the prostate is the closest men have to a Pap for initial screening, but this only checks for enlargement and/or nodulation. By the time there is nodulation or enlargement, the disease process has been fulminating for some time. Pap smears, on the other hand, screen for microscopic changes in the cells of the cervix. In that way women are lucky. They can and should be screened at least once a year and thus they can be warned when an otherwise Hidden Evil is creating minimal to moderate dysplasia. Men, on the other hand, due to their anatomy, have as yet no comparable screening test.[1] Therefore, men, who must be equally infected with HPV as are their female sexual partners, are living largely unaware of this pathogen lurking within them.

It is my clinical impression that there has been a significant increase in the incidence of CIN in the older members of the Baby Boom generation. By this I mean women currently in their late 30s and early to mid 40s. It is exactly these same women who were in the vanguard of the sexual revolution, and it is likewise their male counterparts who tangoed with them. Therefore, it is my hypothesis that there will be an epidemic of prostate problems, including cancer, in the next 10-15 years amongst men who are now in their late 30s and early 40s. This hypothesis is based on the fact that the prostate and cervix are the same tissue embryologically and, therefore, might tend to react similarly or analogously to a single pathogen. HPV has been implicated in cases of bladder cancer.[2] As part of the urogenital tract, it is not unreasonable to suspect HPV might also reach the prostate to cause pathogenesis there.

Anne M. Haywood, MD, writing in *The New England Journal of Medicine*, states:

> What is currently known about persistent viral infections probably represents just the tip of the iceberg. Indirect evidence suggests that the primary cause of a wide variety of diseases may be persistent viral infection.[3]

Dr. Haywood goes on to list the viruses known to produce persistent infections in humans. These include:

Rubella
Rubeola
Retroviruses
    HTLV-I
    HTLV-II
    HIV (HTLV-III)
Herpesviruses
    Cytomegalvirus (CMV)
    Epstein-Barr virus (EBV)
    Herpes simplex I & II (HSV I & II)
    Herpes zoster

Papovaviruses
    Polymaviruses
    Papillomaviruses
Adenoviruses
Hepatitis B
"Unconventional viruses"
    Kuru agent
    Cruetzfeldt-Jacob disease agent

Further, Dr. Haywood lists the diseases postulated by Western researchers caused by persistent viral infections:

Neurological diseases
    Multiple Sclerosis (MS)
    Amyotrophic Lateral Sclerosis (ALS)
    Parkinson's disease
    Presenile dementia (Alzheimer's disease)
    Schizophrenia
    Depressive disease
Neoplasms
Birth defects
Crohn's Disease
Autoimmune diseases
    Systemic Lupus Erythmatosus (SLE)
    Rheumatoid arthritis (RA)
    Dermomyositis
    Periarteritis nodosa
Diabetes
Paget's disease
Miscellaneous endocrine deficits

According to Dr. Haywood, HPV is one of the viruses known to cause persistent infections in humans and such persistent infections are suspected as a contributory etiology in the formation of neoplasms, such as benign prostatic hypertrophy and prostate cancer. Dr. Haywood states,

> The viruses that have been found to be associated with malignant disease in humans include HTLV-I, HTLV-II, Epstein-Barr virus, hepatitis B, and some types of papillomaviruses ... In patients with immune deficiencies, oncogenesis may be facilitated.[4]

The embryological correlation between the cervix and the prostate lies in the anatomical junction they share. Ectoderm and endoderm reunite in the external os of the cervix and the prostatic utricle. In the fertilized ovum, two cell types differentiate into a single-cell layer called the endoderm and a proliferating layer called ectoderm. Proliferating cells, called the mesoderm, which differentiate from the ectoderm separate these two cell types except at two places -- 1) the cloaca where the anus, urethra, and vagina later open and 2) the bucopharyngeal membrane which becomes the mouth and lips.

The endoderm in the adult becomes the one-cell lining of all the organs and glands which embryologically develop from the alimentary canal: the thyroid, parathyroid, thymus, liver, pancreas, respiratory tract, eustachian tube, middle ear, inner tympanic membrane, antrum, mastoid air cells, bladder (except the trigone), distal urethra, greater vestibular glands and vagina, and the bulbourethral glands and the glands of the prostate.

The ectoderm invaginates along the central axis to become at first the primitive streak. Then the neural plate appears which eventually becomes the central nervous system. Externally, the ectoderm forms the epidermis, nails, hair, epithelium of the sebaceous sweat glands, mammary glands, and mucous lining of the mouth, nose, and paranasal sinuses. As the ectoderm proliferates, every other structure of the body develops.

The embryonic mesoderm derives from this ectodermal layer. It fills all the spaces between the ectoderm and endoderm except at the cloaca and bucopharyngeal membranes. The bilaminar embryo becomes trilaminar with the spread of this third tissue which gives rise to three further subdivisions of tissue: the lateral mesoderm, the intermediate mesoderm, and the paraxial mesoderm. It is these three embryonic tissues which give rise to the suprarenal cortex, the sinovial membranes, lymph vessel walls and lymphatic tissue, blood vessel walls and blood cells, smooth, voluntary, and cardiac muscle, cartilage, bone, and all other connective tissue.

The intermediate mesoderm becomes many parts of the urogenital system. It forms two columns of tissue from the septum transversum to third lumbar vertebra. The blood supply of the glomerular ductules comes off the aorta. The mesonephric duct remains in adults as the duct of the epididymus, ductus deferens, ejaculatory duct, prostatic urethra distal to the utricle, and the uretic portion of the bladder in the male; while, in the female, it remains as the urethra, uretic portion of the bladder, and the vestigial duct of the epoophoron and paroophoron.

The paramesonephric ducts develop in the mesonephros. They meet in the midline to form in women the uterus and the fallopian tubes and, in the male, the appendix of the testes and prostatic utricle.

In men, the endoderm of the cloaca folds in to form the urogenital sinus. The paramesonephric ducts touch the wall of this invagination and a thickened plate of cells develops until the two original tissue types reunite. The prostatic utricle is thus comprised of the endoderm of the urogenital sinus and the lining of the epithelium of the mesonephric and paramesonephric ducts. Whereas, in women, within the cervical canal, the urogenital sinus epithelium of the vagina interfaces with the solid epithelium of the paramesonephric ducts of the uterus. This interface is the cervix.

I believe that Traditional Chinese Medicine likewise recognizes the identity of the uterine cervix and the prostate. The *Bao Gong* is literally the Wrapper Palace. However, in everyday parlance, it refers to the Uterus. Nonetheless, it is said in Chinese medicine that, "The *Bao Gong* is the place where body Essence is concealed and, therefore, both sexes are endowed with it."[5] Chen Zhi-duo felt that, "The only difference between male and female is that it has a narrowly shaped upper part with a base in females and a prolonged and equally narrowed form in males."[6] Kathleen Belko, DC and Dipl. Ac., believes the sinu-utricular cord is the "prolonged and ... narrowed" structure in men which dilates into the 6 mm utricle.[7] This structure is analogously similar to the uterus and its neck. Zhang Jing-yue stated that, "Both the Essence and Blood of both sexes converge in this Organ (*Bao Gong*)."[8] While Tang Zong-hai further stated that, "The alternative name for the female *Bao Gong vis a vis* menstruation and reproduction is the Sea of Blood (*Xue Hai*); while the male equivalent is the *Dan Tian, Qi Hai,* or *Jing She* (Chamber of Essence)..."[9]

This Chamber of Essence or *Jing She* is the prostate or, perhaps more specifically, the prostatic utricle. The traditional Chinese name for the cervix is the *Bao Men* or the Gate of the *Bao (Gong)*. Another name or description is the *Zi Gong Kou* or mouth to the Fetal Palace. As such, it is conceived of as part of the *Bao Gong* and not some separate Organ.

There are over 1 million cases of HPV infection *reported* per year in the United States.[10] This means one reported case per 200 Americans *per year*. If HPV can remain hidden indefinitely and often is asymptomatic, that means that there are an awful lot of men infected who may be in for a rude awakening as age takes its natural toll on their *Jing* Essence.

WESTERN ETIOLOGIES OF PROSTATE CANCER

In modern Western medicine, the etiology of prostate cancer is not clear-cut. Dr. E. David Crawford, professor and chairman of the Division of Urology at the University of Colorado Health Sciences Center, states:

> Although no single factor has been shown to be directly related to the cause of prostate cancer, genetic, hormonal, and environmental factors all have been strongly implicated as a cause. In order to develop prostate cancer, there are two prerequisites, besides being male. The first is the presence of testosterone and the second is

time.[11]

Leaving aside for the moment testosterone's role in prostate cancer, some researchers feel that essentially all men develop prostate cancer with age. Because this cancer grows so slowly, most men die of other causes before they die of prostate cancer. As Dr. Crawford says:

> Prostate cancer is common in men over the age of 50 and, in fact, increases in incidence from the fifth through the ninth decades of life. As many as 70 to 80 percent of men in their ninth decade will be found to have areas of prostate cancer is their glands are examined carefully.[12]

Jack Finch, researcher for the Central Cancer Registry, State of Colorado, says that autopsies on men over 50 years of age support the thesis that almost if not all men over that age do have cancerous lesions in their prostate. According to Mr. Finch, 85% of male autopsies over a certain age reveal prostate cancer. This goes along with my hypothesis that HPV and similar viruses may cause prostate cancer and are, in Traditional Chinese Medicine, Hidden Evils. They may remain hidden for long periods of time but tend to become active with age and the natural consumption and, therefore, decline of *Jing*. This also goes along with the higher incidence of condyloma in men after the seventh decade of life. As the *Nei Jing* states, the *Jing* becomes exhausted in men at 8x8 or 64 years of age.

Dr. Crawford goes on to say:

> Family history plays a role in that prostate cancer is more common in a son whose father has prostate cancer. Other risk factors include lower socio-economic status, increased sexual

activity, marriage, and a history of sexually transmitted disease.[12]

Inherited tendencies towards prostate cancer may be explained in TCM terms as a predisposition towards more Heat constitutionally and/or less Kidney Yin or *Jing*. Either of these tendencies may predispose a person to the flourishing of a *Wen Xie* or Warm Evil. In addition to a constitutional dyscrasia of Yang *vis a vis* Yin, it is also possible that an inherited tendency to prostate cancer is due to *Tai Du* or Fetal Toxins. These are *Du* or Toxins passed from either parent to the zygote at the moment of conception or generated during gestation due to the mother's diet or disease. Typically, these *Tai Du*, when they manifest, do so as *Wen Bing* arising from the *Xue Fen* and moving from Inside to Outside, such as measles, chicken pox, and infantile eczema. This concept of *Tai Du* in many ways is quite similar to the homeopathic concept of miasms or inherited tendencies to disease.

Lower socio-economic status can imply a wide range of disease causing factors: poor nutrition, emotional stress, increased use of alcohol and drugs, careless sexual hygiene, lack of medical screening and care, poor health education, overwork, and/or increased, multi-partner sexual activity. However, when STD (sexually transmitted disease) researchers use the words "lower socio-economic status", they assume that early sexual activity and multiple sexual partners is part of that definition.[14] Inner city, poor children typically become sexually active at 12 years of age.[15]

Increased sexual activity, marriage, and a history of sexually transmitted disease are all more revealing. Increased sexual activity can mean either more sex with a single partner or more different partners. If Dr. Crawford means more sex with the same partner, this may imply increased expenditures of *Jing* Essence. If it means more sexual partners, which, realistically,

I think is implied, this suggests a venereal transmission. At first sight, marriage would seem to contradict the idea of venereal transmission. However, many married couples do not use condoms since they assume their monogamy protects them from venereal disease. However, most men and many, if not most women have sex with other than their spouses either before or during marriage. Many men and women both may be infected with HPV and not know it. Leaving aside the question of who infected whom, men, assuming no need to use protection with their wives, may be being infected or reinfected with mutating strains of virus in their marriage bed.

As for a history of STD, this suggests the likelihood of HPV infection as well. On the one hand, any venereal disease will compromise the immune system in general and also imbalance the Lower Burner predisposing it towards Dampness and Heat. Therefore, even if HPV and HSV II have not piggy-backed along with gonorrhea, syphilis, or chlamydia, a history of these venereal diseases make one potentially more susceptible to these viruses. Also, a history of venereal disease suggests multiple sexual partners and an inattention to sexual hygiene.

THE WESTERN DIAGNOSIS OF PROSTATITIS, PROSTATIC HYPERTROPHY, & PROSTATE CANCER

Western medicine divides prostate disease into 3 broad categories: prostatitis, benign prostatic hypertrophy, and prostate cancer.

Prostatitis

Prostatitis means inflammation of the prostate. It is subdivided into 3 distinct types in Western medicine.

Acute bacterial prostatitis is an acute infection of the prostate. Its signs and symptoms are fever and chills, urinary frequency and urgency, perineal and low back pain, varying degrees of difficulty and obstruction when urinating, nocturia, and often arthralgia or joint pain and/or myalgia or muscle pain. There may also be hematuria. Digital rectal examination reveals a tender, swollen, and indurated gland which is usually warm to the touch. Culture of the prostatic secretion yields large numbers of pathogenic bacteria.

Chronic bacterial prostatitis may manifest a diverse group of symptoms. Its hallmark is relapsing urinary tract infections due to the same pathogenic bacteria residing in the prostatic secretions. Some patients are asymptomatic. However, most experience low back and perineal pain and urinary urgency and frequency. Typically there is dysuria as well. If infection has spread to the scrotum, there will be intense, localized pain, swelling, redness, and severe tenderness to palpation. Digital rectal exam reveals a moderately tender and irregularly indurated or boggy gland. Definitive diagnosis of chronic bacterial prostatitis is made by microscopic inspection of cultures of prostatic secretions.

Chronic nonbacterial prostatitis' signs and symptoms are essentially the same as above. However, these patients rarely have a history of urinary tract infection, and microscopic inspection of cultures fail to reveal pathogenic bacteria. I have found that some men with the above signs and symptoms of chronic nonbacterial prostatitis experience these as the prodromal signs and symptoms of an HSV II outbreak. Most cases of prostatitis are, in fact, this third kind -- chronic nonbacterial prostatitis. Western medicine considers its etiologies or cause unknown but my experience suggests a venereally transmitted, viral etiology.

Benign Prostatic Hypertrophy

Benign prostatic hypertrophy (BPH) refers to an adenomatous hyperplasia of the paraurethral prostate gland or that part of the gland which surrounds the urethra. It is a common condition in men over the age of 50 and causes variable degrees of urinary obstruction. According to Western medicine, the cause or etiology of benign prostatic hypertrophy is unknown, but it is suspected that the aging process, with its shifts in relative hormone levels, has something to do with this. Since hormones play such a large role in the immune response, this also suggests that due to hormonal fluctuations commensurate with aging, some pathogen which formerly had been latent has been allowed to become active, i.e. a *Fu Wen Xie*. The signs and symptoms of benign prostatic hypertrophy include bladder outlet obstruction resulting in progressive urinary frequency and nocturia, hesitancy and intermittency of stream, decreased size and force of the stream, sensations of incomplete emptying, terminal dribbling, almost continuous over-flow dribbling, or complete urinary retention. Digital rectal examination may be misleading with the size of the prostate being relatively normal.

Sometimes, benign prostatic hypertrophy may be complicated by hematuria, burning with urination, and fever and chills if there is concomitant urinary tract infection (UTI). Episodes of acute urinary retention may follow prolonged attempts to hold the urine, exposure to cold, immobilization, or drinking alcohol. A distended bladder may be palpated externally. Prolonged urinary retention, either partial or complete, may eventually result in renal failure and uremia.

Prostate Cancer

There are 2 broad categories of prostate cancer: adenocarcinoma and sarcoma of the prostate. Adenocarcinoma of the prostate is the most common malignancy in men over 65 and sarcoma of the prostate is rarely encountered in children. Undifferentiated prostatic carcinoma and squamous cell carcinoma of the prostate are variants of adult adenocarcinoma.

Prostate cancer is very slow to progress and often remains asymptomatic for a long period of time. During its later stages, there may be bladder outlet obstruction, hematuria, and pyuria or pus in the urine. Metastases to the pelvis and lumbar spine may cause bone pain. Digital rectal exam may reveal stony, hard indurations, but these are not pathognomic since they may also occur in granulomatous prostatitis, prostatic tuberculosis, prostatic calculi, and other, more unusual prostate diseases. A firm and nodularly irregular prostate is pathognomic which later exhibits extension of induration and fixation of the gland to the rectum and lateral pelvic walls.

Currently, digital rectal examination is the preferred method for screening for and diagnosing prostate cancer at an early stage. However, digital rectal exam still fails to detect all cases of prostate cancer. At the moment, newer methods of diagnosis are being explored. These include transrectal ultrasound and a blood test called prostatic specific antigen (PSA). Western medicine recommends that all men over 45 years of age begin getting regularly scheduled (once per year) digital rectal exams to screen for prostate cancer the same way that it recommends all women over 40 receive regularly scheduled mammograms to screen for breast cancer.

Similar to the staging of cervical disorders, there does exist a classification system in Western medicine for the severity of prostate cancer. There are four stages identified as A through D.

Stage A is defined as the incidental finding of prostate cancer in a patient undergoing a transurethral resection of his prostate for an otherwise presumed benign prostatic hypertrophy. Digital rectal exam prior to surgery fails to evidence any hard nodulations on the gland.

Stage B refers to a cancerous patient in whom a nodule was found during a routine physical exam including a digital rectal exam.

Stage C refers to a patient who has tumors spread locally through the prostate capsule and involving surrounding structures.

Stage D means that cancer originating in the prostate has now spread to the adjacent lymph nodes or bones.

Dr. Crawford states that, "Unfortunately, 50 to 70 percent of patients whom we see with prostate cancer have either locally advanced or metastatic disease."[16] This is because 1) as yet, relatively few men avail themselves of routine digital rectal exams, 2) these exams still only identify diseased patients after there has been considerable neoplastic activity, and 3) this disease develops asymptomatically, i.e. hiddenly.

THE WESTERN MEDICAL TREATMENT OF PROSTATE PROBLEMS

Both acute and chronic bacterial prostatitis are treated by antibiotics. If there is complete urinary retention, this may be remedied by urethral catheterization or punch suprapubic cystostomy. The latter is the inserting of a drainage tube into the bladder above the pubic bone. Western medicine has no effective treatment for chronic nonbacterial prostatitis and considers this a very recalcitrant and difficult disease. This recalcitrance to treatment also supports my hypothesis that it is a viral disease.

Benign prostatic hypertrophy is treated by catheterization, either urethral or suprapubic, until transurethral prostatic resection can be done. This last procedure is popularly referred to as a "ream job" if it is done through the urethral opening without incision. Larger benign prostates may be surgically operated on suprapubically, retropubically, or perineally. Although morbidity and mortality are low, this surgery may result in permanent impotence and/or incontinence.

For localized prostate cancer, standard Western medicine depends on two treatment options. These are surgery and radiation. Western medicine considers both of these as effective treatments which offer "excellent long-term control and survival",[17] with radical prostatectomy being the treatment of choice. However, both procedures usually result in impotence and urinary incontinence. Recently, a surgical procedure has been developed which preserves the nerves necessary for erection.

However, most prostate cancer patients have either localized advanced or metastatic disease which are not curable with current, conventional Western medical treatment. Because testosterone is required for this cancer to grow, Western medicine recommends several methods which interrupt this male hormone, including bilateral orchiectomy or surgical castration. Female hormones, central hormone inhibitors, such as leuprolide, and anti-androgens are also used. But, the bottom line at this time in patients with advanced and metastatic prostate cancer is that, "Regardless of the form of therapy utilized, patients eventually fail."[18]

CHAPTER EIGHT
TRADITIONAL CHINESE MEDICINE & PROSTATE PROBLEMS

Similar to cervical dysplasia, there is no classical Chinese disease category which corresponds exactly to either prostatitis, benign prostatic hypertrophy, or prostate cancer. Nor is there in the current English literature a *Bian Zheng* description of the differential diagnosis of prostate problems or differentiation of Patterns. *Long Bi* means urinary retention or difficulty. This term is used to cover benign prostatic hypertrophy as evidenced by its use thus in *Acupuncture Case Histories From China*.[1] However, *Long Bi* can also describe urinary retention due to other reasons as well.

In Chinese medicine, there is also a classification of urinary disorders called the *Wu Lin* or Five *Lin*. *Lin* literally means dripping and so the *Wu Lin* are five different kinds of urinary dribbling or dripping disease. However, most Western translators prefer to translate this category as the Five Urinary Disturbances or Urinary Stranguries. These five are:

Shi Lin	Stone *Lin*
Qi Lin	Qi (Stagnation) *Lin*
Xue Lin	Blood *Lin*, i.e. hematuria accompanying strangury
Re Lin	Heat or Hot *Lin*

Lao Lin   Fatigue or Exhaustion *Lin*

As a group, the *Wu Lin* cover everything in Western medicine from cystitis to nephrolithiasis, including prostatitis, benign prostatic hypertrophy, and prostate cancer. In addition to this five-fold classification, there are also *Sha Lin* or Sandy *Lin*, referring to urinary gravel, and *Zhuo Lin* or Turbid *Lin*. *Zhuo Lin* refers to turbid, milky, or cloudy urination and can also cover prostatitis.

Other classical Chinese terms which cover various symptoms associated with prostate conditions include *Jing Sou Bu Li*, difficulty urinating; *Sou Shuo*, frequent micturition; and *Xiao Bian Liu Li*, dribbling urination.

Based on an analysis of two modern Chinese patent medicines for prostatitis (Jie Jie Wan, aka Kai Kit Wan, and Qian Lie Xian Wan) and on my personal clinical experience, I think I can say that the TCM disease mechanisms associated with prostatitis, prostatic hypertrophy, and prostate cancer other than or in addition to External Invasion through venereal transmission of a *Fu Wen Xie* are:

>Damp Heat Accumulating in the Bladder
>Liver Congestion/Qi Stagnation
>Stagnant Blood
>Kidney Deficiency

The first 3 of these mechanisms occur more in middle-aged men and the last is more prominent in older patients. As in cervical dysplasia, it is the inter-relationship of these four factors creating the background environment plus the presence of a *Fu Wen Xie* which I worry about causing a marked increase or earlier development of prostate problems in male Baby Boomers. Although I have no proof that viral infection complicates all or even most current cases of prostate disease, whether benign or malignant, I do think it likely that viral infection will play a part in these diseases in the near future.

Damp Heat Accumulating in the Bladder

Damp Heat Accumulating in the Bladder can be due to both dysfunction of the Spleen and Kidneys in transporting and transforming Water. If Damp percolates down from the Spleen, it is usually due to faulty diet, including too many Damp foods, Cold foods, and too copious and cold liquids drunk with meals. This may be aggravated by worry and overwork. If Evil Dampness accumulates in the Lower Burner due to faulty Kidney Qi function, this is mostly the result of aging, sexual fatigue (*Fang Lao*), and the Kidneys' natural decline. Dampness obstructing the flow of Qi in the Lower Burner may generate Heat and thus give rise to Damp Heat. In addition, Heat from Depressive Liver Fire or a Hot Liver may become entangled with Dampness also engendering Damp Heat. Further, Heat itself may steam the Juices causing a condensation of Dampness and thus Damp Heat. All of these mechanisms can be aggravated by eating Damp Hot foods, such as alcohol and spicy, greasy, fried foods, beef, and pork.

Liver Congestion/Qi Stagnation

Liver Qi Congestion may result in both Heat and Dampness accumulating in the Lower Burner. Since Qi is Yang, if it accumulates due to Stagnation past a certain point, it will transform into Evil Heat. Since Qi transports Water, if the Qi is stuck or sluggish, this may allow Dampness to accumulate. However, Liver Qi can result simply in difficult or retarded urination for the same reason without necessarily having to include accumulation of Damp Heat in the diagnosis. This is the mechanism behind *Qi Lin* or Qi Dribbling. In *Qi Lin*, urination becomes difficult proportionate to the amount of emotional stress and, therefore, the impatency of Liver Qi. In our culture at least, a certain amount of Liver Qi seems universal amongst urban and suburban Baby Boomers.

Stagnant Blood

Stagnant Blood is a common complicating factor in patients with prostate problems, whether benign or malignant. This is *not* based on digital rectal exam finding nodes or hypertrophy but is based primarily on tongue and pulse signs and symptoms. I have italicized the not in the preceding sentence to emphasize the fact that in TCM every palpable lump is not automatically or necessarily Stagnant Blood and especially not so if the lump cannot be palpated from the outside of the body. Typically, this Stagnant Blood is due to long-term obstruction due to any or all of Stagnant Qi, Stagnant Heat, or Stagnant Dampness. It is usually not due to traumatic injury. There is a tendency to develop Stagnant Blood with age in any case due to the decline of Qi and Blood, and Lower Burner circulation in particular easily becomes or is inherently a little sluggish. In our culture, this is aggravated by our sedentary lifestyle.

In Asia, prostate problems are sometimes referred to colloquially as Buddhist monk disease since Buddhist monks typically spend a lot of time sitting. It is my personal experience that often when I begin a meditation retreat, I experience after a few days some hemorrhoidal discomfort due to Stagnation. In celibate monks, this Stagnation is compounded by lack of discharge of Stagnation by orgasmic release.

Dampness, Heat, Stagnant Qi, and Stagnant Blood are all mutually inter-promoting. The first three are common dyscrasias in middle-aged males. Over time, Stagnant Blood then tends to develop.

Kidney Deficiency

Kidney Deficiency refers to Kidney Qi *vis a vis* urination. It is the Kidney Qi which governs the transportation and transformation of Water in the Lower Burner. Kidney Deficiency is differentiated into Kidney Yang Deficiency and Kidney Yin Deficiency. Both of these Patterns are accompanied by urinary disturbances. However, in each case, frequency, nocturia, enuresis, and incontinence are specifically due to insufficient Kidney Qi transporting and transforming Liquids.

In Kidney Yang Deficiency, there is insufficient Heat to transform Liquids. In Yin Deficiency there is too much Heat which over-transforms Liquids. However, in both cases, there is insufficient Qi to hold Liquids at first and to propel Liquids finally. As everyone ages, first Kidney Yin becomes Deficient and then, eventually, Kidney Yang becomes Deficient. When both Yin and Yang become Deficient, then we can speak of Kidney *Jing* Deficiency, the *Jing* Essence depending upon the correct inter-relationship between Yin and Yang.

Because Kidney Qi Deficiency is identical to old age, this also explains why prostate problems are most often a geriatric condition. However, Kidney Qi Deficiency prostate diseases are usually complicated by elements of Dampness, Heat, and Stagnation of Qi and Blood engendered or initiated during middle-age. Although these mechanisms are typically deemed adequate in contemporary TCM to account for a cancerous condition, cancers themselves are usually also described as being Toxic as well. I believe the source of Toxins in many, if not all, prostate cancers is a venereally transmitted *Li Qi* or *Fu Wen Xie* -- in Western terms, a virus, either HPV or HSV II, both together, or some other virus as yet unidentified.

Testosterone

Above we mentioned that the presence of testosterone was one of the factors Western medicine has identified as being necessary for the development of prostate cancer. TCM theory can shed some light on this as well. Testosterone is a male sex hormone manufactured and secreted by the testicles. The testes are called the *Wai Shen* in Chinese medicine. This means the Outer Kidneys. This name underscores the testes' being part of the Chinese *Shen* or Kidneys. Testosterone is an Internal Secretion related to the Yang aspect of the Kidneys. Therefore, functionally, it is part of the *Ming Men Zhi Huo*. It is the *Ming Men* which supplies the Righteous Heat of the Lower Burner. It is also this Righteous Heat which, if Excessive or Congested, can give rise to internally generated Evil Heat. This Heat can also be transferred to any other pathologic Accumulation, such as Dampness or Stagnant Blood. And, additionally, flourishing *Ming Men* Fire can exacerbate any Externally-invading Hot pathogen.

The *Ming Men* Fire is, *vis a vis* the Kidneys, essentially the same as Kidney Yang or Kidney Fire. The process of life is the consumption and transformation of Yin substance by the Fire of Life. This Fire of Life consumes and transforms the *Yin Jing* producing all the myriad functions of life. Therefore, Yin Essence is consumed by Yang Fire as one lives, and, as one ages, there arises a relative Excess of Heat compared to Yin substance. This relative Yang Excess attendant with older middle-age and the beginning of old age is responsible for most strokes, heart attacks, hypertension, menopausal complaints in women, and senile insomnia. It also helps explain why prostate problems tend to arise after the age of 40.

If we posit that testosterone is functionally a part of the *Ming Men Zhi Huo* and that the *Ming Men* is intimately connected with the Heat that Chinese medicine says is almost always part of prostate conditions at middle-age, then the necessity of testosterone in the development of prostate problems is understandable. Based on the relationship between prostate problems and testosterone and the fact that testosterone is produced in the testes, it is also understandable why Western medicine often recommends castration as part of the treatment of prostate cancer.

Typically, when a male animal is castrated, there will be a tendency for it to gain weight and to become both less active in general and less aggressive in particular. In Chinese medicine, this tendency is described as being due to less of the Yang Fire of Life. Therefore, both form and behavior become more Yin. In terms of Chinese disease categorization, Warm Evils are, because they are Hot, Yang. With but a few exceptions, anything, including testosterone, which makes a person Hotter internally may initiate or accelerate a Hidden Warm Evil to become active and flourish.

THE TCM DIAGNOSIS OF PROSTATE PROBLEMS

Diagnosis in contemporary Chinese TCM is typically tripartite. First there is the statement of the Western disease category established by Western diagnostic standards and procedures. Secondly, there is the statement of traditional Chinese disease category, such as *Zhuo Lin, Long Bi,* or *Lao Lin.* These two taken together are referred to as diagnosis by *Bian Bing* or the discrimination of named disease categories. Third, there is the TCM diagnosis based on the discrimination of Patterns. In Chinese, this is called diagnosis by *Bian Zheng.* It is diagnosis by *Bian Zheng* which individualizes a particular patient's case and allows for individualized, holistic treatment. The following are the TCM *Zheng* most commonly associated with prostate problems.

Damp Heat in the Bladder

The signs and symptoms of Damp Heat in the Bladder are frequency and urgency of urination, difficult urination, and burning pain in the urethra with urination. If Dampness predominates, the urine will be turbid or cloudy. If Heat predominates, there will be more burning and pain and there may be hematuria. The textbook description of the tongue is red with a yellow coating. Often there is a yellow, greasy coating at the root of the tongue. The pulse is generally rapid. The *Chi* position is often deep and typically wiry. In some cases, the pulse may be slippery and wiry or fine and wiry. If the pulse is fine and wiry, this means Dampness has impeded the Spleen's ability to *Sheng Hua* or create and transform the Blood.

Liver Congestion/Qi Stagnation

Liver Qi Stagnation is evidenced by pain preceding the flow of urination, lower abdominal cramping and/or distention, a normal, slightly *Qing* colored tongue, a wiry pulse, and a tendency for urination to become particularly difficult or obstructed due to emotional stress. The *Chi* position is characteristically deep. This deepness is due to the problem being Internal as opposed to a Kidney Deficiency Pattern.

Blood Stagnation

Blood Stagnation typically manifests as piercing, stabbing pain, ecchymotic patches or a more significantly purple tongue, and a deep, astringent, possibly irregular, and almost always wiry pulse. Pain worsens at night. If there is hematuria, the Blood is dark in color and may contain clots.

Kidney Deficiency

The signs and symptoms of Kidney Deficiency are polyuria, nocturia, dribbling urination, weak stream, or retention of urine accompanied by weakness of the lumbar region and knee joints. If Kidney Yin is Deficient, the urine will be scant in amount and yellow in color. There will be signs and symptoms of Deficiency Heat rising above, such as tinnitus, palpitations, and Heat in the Five Centers. The pulse will be fine and rapid, or, in older patients, flooding and floating. The tongue is red, possibly cracked, and has a scant coating. If Kidney Yang is Deficient, there will be pallor, fear of cold, desire for warm food and drinks, a pale tongue with white coating, and a deep, thready, weak, and possibly even slow pulse.

These symptom/sign pictures are simple, idealized, textbook descriptions. Most real-life patients will be some combination of the above signs and symptoms making a composite picture of several or even all of the above Patterns. In addition, concurrent dyscrasias in other Organs may further complicate any individual's personal Pattern, such as Heart/Small Intestine Fire transferred to the Bladder, Stomach Heat, Spleen/Small Intestine Deficiency, and Lung Deficiency or Lung Heat to name several commonly encountered complications. In such real-life situations, the practitioner simply parses out each sign and symptom gathered by the Four (Methods) of diagnosis and analyzes them according to the disease mechanism logic of TCM.

As far as diagnosing an External invading Hidden Warm Evil, this must be based primarily on questioning, although the penis may be examined for visible venereal warts or a ViraPap test can be done. If a man has prostatitis, benign prostatic hypertrophy, or prostate cancer and has venereal warts, a history of herpes genitalia, a history of having had unprotected sex with a woman known to have had cervical dysplasia or cervical cancer, or has had multiple sexual partners, *Fu Wen Xie* involvement should be considered.

As of this writing, I know of no definitive diagnostic method for determining the presence of a *Fu Wen Xie* according to the classical Four (Methods of) diagnosis of Chinese medicine if that Evil is truly hidden and, therefore, asymptomatic. Although a *Fu Mai* or hidden pulse is classically indicative of a *Fu Xie*, many patients have *Fu Xie* without having a *Fu Mai*. For some *Fu Wen Xie*, such as HIV, EBV, and CMV, blood tests can be done. For HPV in women, there is the ViraPap. For men, there is also the ViraPap, but this is as yet expensive and not widely available. Therefore, the method I use for determining asymptomatic or hidden viral infection beyond questioning is Vega biokinesiology (VBK). As mentioned above, using potentitized resonance filters made from HPV nosodes, it is possible to test for and confirm the presence of viruses, such as HPV, in otherwise asymptomatic men.

CHAPTER NINE
THE PREVENTIVE TREATMENT OF PROSTATE PROBLEMS

As a TCM gynecologist, I have little personal experience in treating prostate disease. I have treated several men over the past 10 years, a couple successfully and one unsuccessfully. If a patient already has an established Western medical diagnosis of a benign prostate problem, Chinese medicine, including herbs and acupuncture, should be tried. In cases of known prostate cancer, some combination of Western medicine, both conventional and alternative, and Chinese medicine should probably be used. Such a combination should at least palliate the discomfort and increase both the quality and length of life.

However, the main impetus of this section of this book is to recommend to young and middle-aged American males who are infected with HPV and HSV II to seek early, preventive care. *This includes any man who has had unprotected sex with a woman who has had a positive Pap and any man after 40 years of age.* My suggestions for my fellow men parallel those for women who have had a positive Pap smear at some time in their life and are now in remission. Even if HPV and/or HSV II turn out not to be involved in prostate problems and especially prostate cancer, because of the almost universal incidence of prostate problems in older men, most of the preventive regimes given herein do make sense no matter what the Western etiology.

The key points in the prevention of the activation of a *Fu Wen Xie* are maintenance of abundant *Jing* Essence and minimization of accumulation of Dampness and Heat in the Lower Burner. As we have seen above, Dampness and Heat almost always play a part in the disease mechanism of prostate problems. These two basic issues -- maintenance of *Jing* and elimination of Damp Heat -- can be addressed through diet, exercise, deep relaxation, herbal therapy, orthomolecular therapy, homotoxicology, acupuncture, massage, and sexual pacing.

DIET

First of all, one should minimize or eliminate foods which are Damp, Hot, aggravate the Liver, or weaken the Kidneys. This includes over-eating of meats, spicy foods, greasy foods, fried, broiled, and charred foods, alcohol, and coffee. One should also avoid over-eating in general. Secondly, if there is any suspicion of candidiasis, an anti-candida regime should be implemented as described above. And third, maintenance of good Large Intestine function should be stressed long-term due to its relationship to *Wei Qi* and Kidney Yang. Colon-cleansing has likewise been described above. A corollary of diet is the complete avoidance of recreational drugs which plunder the Yin, exhaust the *Jing*, and inflame Deficiency Heat.

EXERCISE

Regular aerobic exercise 3 times per week for 20 consecutive minutes per session should be considered *de rigueur* for most middle-aged men. Such aerobic exercise blows off or exteriorizes Heat, circulates the Qi and Blood, and, therefore, aids in the transportation and transformation of Fluids. When a person nears 55 or 60, Chinese medicine often suggests less strenuous forms of exercise, such as *Qi Gong* and *Tai Ji*

Chuan, so as not to dissipate unnecessarily Righteous Qi. This is somewhat subject to individual constitution and condition. However, even after 60, some form of regular exercise is vitally important for the maintenance of good health. In general, we should all walk and ride bicycles whenever we can, climb stairs instead of using elevators, and regularly rise from our desks to move about, stretch, and circulate our Qi and Blood.

DEEP RELAXATION

Regular, programmed, deep relaxation is one of the best, if not the very best way to abort Liver Qi and Heat derived from Depressive Liver Fire. In addition, surplus Qi and Blood produced Postnatally are converted into Acquired Essence during periods of deep relaxation and sleep. As mentioned above, proper amounts of relaxation and exercise together promote sound sleep, abundant energy, good digestion and elimination, and mental equipose. All of these add up to more Acquired Essence and less Evil Heat.

HERBAL THERAPY

There are two divisions to herbal therapy for the prevention of prostate problems. First are suggestions for men who know or strongly suspect they are infected with at least one venereally transmitted virus. This includes men with known genital herpes and genital warts and men who have had unprotected sex with a woman with a history of CIN. To clarify this last criterion, this means a woman who either had cervical dysplasia before one's sexual encounter or developed dysplasia or cervical cancer at some point after one's *liaison*. As mentioned above, it is possible to test for asymptomatic viral infection using homeopathic nosodes and Vega biokinesiology or electronic Vegatesting. It is also possible for a man to get a ViraPap test and HPV DNA probe screening although this technology is, as yet, not widely available.

1) Suggestions for Men with a Known or Strongly Suspected Viral Infection

Herpes Genitalia

Men with herpes genitalia who have prodromal symptoms before the outbreak of skin lesions can, at the very first hint of an attack, take one of the herbal formulas discussed above as appropriate for prodromal use. These include Health Concerns' Astra Isatis and Qualiherbs' Tang Kuei & Gambir Combination. Health Concerns' Essence Chamber Tablets can also abort an incipient herpes outbreak due to Damp Heat and Stagnation. It will be described in detail further below.

In between attacks, one can take any appropriate formula based on one's constitution and condition to optimize balance in general. However, one should also consider the use of specific anti-viral formulas in addition, such as Health Concerns' Power Mushrooms or Bioradiance distributed by K'an Herbs. Although Bioradiance is, compared to most other herbal medicines, very expensive, I feel that the potential long-term health risks of herpes genitalia justify its use. Bioradiance, described in detail above, is usually taken for only 1 year for herpes. If taken at 40 or 45 years of age, it may help insure another 40 years of good health. As mentioned above, the creator of Bioradiance does believe that it eliminates HPV as well as HSV I & II and, therefore, its use may possibly accomplish both objectives at once.

For the treatments of herpes outbreaks themselves, if the man is relatively robust and his *Bian Zheng* diagnosis is Dampness, Heat, and Hot Toxins, the famous formula Long Dan Xie Gan

Tang (Dragon Gall Liver-draining Decoction) often helps relieve pain, inflammation, and suppuration and shortens the course of the outbreak. This formula has also been described above. It tends to be more suitable for use by men than women since men often have more Qi and Heat. This means their *Bian Zheng* diagnosis is often more simply Excess. This, in turn, means that men can often stand stronger attacking therapy before their Righteous Qi is injured by Cold, Toxin-dissolving ingredients. Other formulas which may be used remedially during an acute herpes outbreak in men are Health Concerns' Coptis Purge Fire Tablets and Isatis Cooling Formula described above.

Genital Warts

Men with either clinical or subclinical genital warts should be treated based on the diagnoses and protocols given in the preceding chapter on anogenital warts. This means that those with clinical warts should be treated with a combination of internally administered and externally applied remedies. While men with subclinical warts should primarily be treated with internal medications.

2) Suggestions for Men without Known or Suspected Viral Infection

For men without known or strongly suspected viral infection, there are still three basic herbal options from which to choose. The first is on-going (or off and on) constitutional therapy based on a discrimination of Dr. Yoo Tae-woo's Three Constitutional Patterns. Dr. Yoo, a famous contemporary Korean doctor, posits 3 basic constitutional dyscrasias. These are called the Yang Excess, Yin Excess, and Kidney Excess Patterns. These Patterns are based on a combination of sophisticated Five Phase and Yin Yang theories. It is Dr.

Yoo's perception that, when one of a *Biao Li* pair becomes Excess, the other typically becomes Deficient.[1] I personally would corroborate this from my clinical practice.

The first Pattern, the Yang Excess constitution, is usually found in robust individuals, most often male, who have a ruddy complexion and a large chest. When young they are mesomorphic, but as they age, they tend to develop large pot-bellies and become endomorphic. In terms of Reichian body-typing, I would say Yang Excess persons tend towards the Psychopathic or mixed Rigid/Psychopathic body type. In this Pattern, the pivotal Organ is the Large Intestine which is Excess. The Lungs, therefore, are Deficient. This leads to a Liver Excess with Spleen Deficiency and Stomach Excess. In addition, the Gallbladder is also Deficient. The Heart and Pericardium are Excess; Small Intestine and Triple Heater Deficient; and the Kidneys are Deficient; while the Bladder is Excess. This leads to an accumulation of Qi under the diaphragm with attendant distention of the upper abdomen and chest. Although the chest is enlarged, these persons do not have good Heart/Lung function. Patients with this constitutional Pattern are typically sore on abdominal palpation at Tian Shu (St 25). In addition, one or more other *Mu* points of the Excess Organs may be sore in individual patients or at specific times.

Yang Excess patients tend to suffer from Hot diseases, including Hot Stagnant Food, Stomach Heat, Liver Yang/Liver Fire Excesses, Damp Heat, Hot Phlegm, Hot Blood, and Stagnant Blood problems. Constitutional therapy designed to regulate the Bowels, activate the Blood, dredge the Liver, clear Heat, transform Phlegm, and eliminate Dampness will help maintain adequate stores of *Jing* and clear and eliminate Heat and Turbidity. A wide variety of herbal formulas may be used depending upon the age of the patient, any current complaints, the season of the year, and the idiosyncratic dyscrasia of the patient revealed by signs and symptoms, the pulse, and especially abdominal palpation. The sorest of the Excess Organ front *Mu* points indicates which of the potentially Excess Organs is most out of balance in a given patient, therefore also implying the most Deficient Organ as well.

Dr. Yoo's second constitutional Pattern is called the Yin Excess Pattern. This is more commonly met amongst obese, pale, atonic females, although it may be encountered amongst males as well. These persons tend to be endomorphic and Masochistic. If the Yang Excess type can be described as beginning as *Shao Yang* and becoming *Tai Yang*, Yin Excess Pattern persons can be described as *Tai Yin*. In this Pattern, Spleen Excess is pivotal with a Deficient Stomach. Da Heng (Sp 15) is pathognomic and will tend to be sore on abdominal palpation. The other Organs which are Excess are the Heart/Pericardium, Gallbladder, Bladder, and Lungs. However, this Excess is Excess Evil Yin, Phlegm Fluids, and Damp Heat. These Excesses are not Excesses of Organ Qi. They are Evil Excesses of pathological substance. The Organs which are Deficient are the Small Intestine, Triple Heater, Liver, Large Intestine, and Kidneys. The Deficiency of these Organ/Bowels is a Deficiency of *Zheng Qi*, Righteous Qi. In particular, the Liver is Liver Blood Deficient and the Kidneys are Kidney Yang Deficient.

Yin Excess patients suffer from an Excess of Yin Evil Accumulation due to Spleen Qi hypofunction *vis a vis* the transportation and transformation of Fluids. Therefore, the central issue is Spleen Dampness. This is, in TCM, a mixed Excess/Deficiency Pattern in which Dr. Yoo has emphasized the Excess aspect. The front *Mu* points of the other typically Excess Organs in this Pattern may be sore to palpation depending upon individual variation and health fluctuations. This patient may develop Damp Heat in the Lower Burner due to poor Spleen function. In addition, since Blood and *Jing* share a common source, this person often does not produce adequate Acquired Essence. These issues can and should be addressed in patients with this Pattern preventively and constitutionally primarily via the Spleen.

Dr. Yoo's third constitutional Pattern is called the Kidney Excess Pattern. These patients tend to be more ectomorphic, although they are often a combination of meso and ectomorphic. They can be either male or female and, according to Reichian body-typing, are usually Rigid if male and Hysteric if female. If they are more pronouncedly ectomorphic, they may also be Oral. This body type can be described in Oriental terms as *Shao Yin*. People with this constitution are of medium build, can be either cerebral or athletic, and tend to be rather highly sexed. Soreness upon palpation at Huang Shu (Ki 16) is confirmatory of this Pattern as is soreness and a lumpy resistance at CV 5-7. Often there is prominent pulsing at or around the umbilicus. The basic mechanism driving this Pattern is a Kidney Yang Excess *vis a vis* Yin. This is called Flaring Ministerial Fire, Flaming Dragon Fire, or Restless Agitation of *Ming Men* Fire in TCM. In this Pattern, which is commonly encountered amongst young and middle-aged Americans, the Kidneys are Excess and so the Bladder is Deficient. The Lungs, Liver, Stomach, Small Intestine, and Triple Heater all also tend to be Excess. While the Large Intestine, Spleen, Heart/Pericardium, and Gallbladder all tend to be Deficient. Flaring *Ming Men* Fire tends to draft up, over-heating the Lungs, Stomach, and Liver. This then scatters the Qi and wastes the Blood and Yin of the Heart making the Spirit restless.

Because the Kidney Excess Pattern is a Yang Excess, I believe two corollaries make men with this Pattern at higher risk for developing prostate cancer. The first is that, since sexual desire is a Yang function of the Kidneys, these men tend to be more sexually active. On the one hand, this suggests more partners and, therefore, more chance of venereal infection.

On the other, it suggests more expenditure of *Jing* Essence. Secondly, Yang Excess suggests a tendency towards Heat from a TCM point of view and higher levels of testosterone from a Western. All of which suggest such men are at greater risk for developing prostate cancer.

The Front *Mu* points associated with the Excess Organs/Bowels may be palpated to assess an individual's specific *Wu Xing/Zang Fu* imbalances and constitutional herbal treatment may be directed at these. Depending upon an individual's momentary, idiosyncratic, dominant Excesses and more obvious Deficiencies, practitioners can choose from a number of formulas. I have written about my personal herbal approach to these three constitutional Patterns elsewhere.[2]

The second herbal option for preventive therapy in men not suspected of viral infection is once or twice yearly courses of Ping Xiao Dan. I have described this formula above under cervical dysplasia. It can be taken for a week at a time, 1-2 times per year by men over 40. Since it helps prevent the arisal of cancers of all types by clearing Heat and dispersing pathologic Accumulations, I think it makes sense prophylactically as long as the man is relatively robust. This is an attacking formula and will harm the Righteous if the Righteous Qi is not in good supply. Therefore, it should not be used too often, for too long, or by persons who are too weak. Even in men with known or strongly suspected viral infection, annual or semi-annual courses of Ping Xiao Dan also make sense.

The third herbal option is to use Essence Chamber Tablets prophylactically in men over 40. I have designed this formula for Health Concerns specifically because of my concern for my own prostate. Essence Chamber Tablets can be used either to treat Damp Heat *Lin* and *Long Bi* or can be taken for 2-4 weeks once or twice per year preventively. They can also be used to abort herpes outbreaks whose prodromal signs and symptoms mimic nonbacterial prostatitis. Essence Chamber Tablets are named for the classical Chinese name for the prostate, the *Jing She*, and are a combination of Western and Chinese herbs. Their ingredients are:

> Herba Larreae Divarticatae
> Radix Hydrangeae Arborscentis
> Fructus Serenoae Serrulatae
> Folium Turnerae Aphrodisiaciae
> Radix Helionadis Dioicae
> Radix Collinsoniae Canadensis
> Sclerotium Poriae Cocoris
> Rhizoma Dioscoreae Hypoglaucae
> Semen Abutilonis Seu Malvae

Herba Larreae Divarticatae is more commonly known as Chaparral. It is Bitter, slightly Acrid, Salty, and Cool. It enters the Liver and Bladder Channels. It is a Heat-clearing, Toxin-dissolving medicinal. Its functions are to clear Heat, dissolve Toxins, and combat cancer. It reduces swellings, eliminates Dampness, and promotes urination. It has demonstrated antiviral effects as well as a long history of empirical use in urinary disturbances. Specifically, Chaparral is effective for the treatment of both genital herpes and warts.

Radix Hydrangeae Arborscentis (Hydrangea) is also a Damp-draining medicinal specific to the treatment of either an inflamed or enlarged prostate. It is Acrid and Cool and enters the Kidney, Bladder, and Large Intestine. It seeps Dampness and promotes urination, clears and eliminates Damp Heat from the Lower Burner, and benefits the separation of Clear and Turbid below. In this formula, Hydrangea assists Chaparral in promoting and smoothing the urination.

Fructus Serenoae Serrulatae (Saw Palmetto Berries) is a *Bu Yang* or Yang tonic ingredient. It is Acrid, Sweet, and Warm and enter the Kidneys, Spleen, and Lungs. It benefits the Kidneys and tonifies the Lungs, thus ensuring the grasping of the Qi sent down by the Lungs. It tonifies the *Wei Qi* and transforms Phlegm due to Kidney Yang Deficiency. In addition, it is also useful in treating Lower Thirsting and Wasting Disease. Like Chaparral and Hydrangea above, they are a specific empirical remedy for enlarged prostate. Saw Palmetto Berries ensure the co-ordinated descension and transformation of Water and adequate Kidney Qi to expel it.

Folium Turnerae Aphrodisiaciae is Damiana. It is another *Bu Yang* herb. It is Acrid and Warm and enters the Liver and Kidneys. It tonifies and activates Yang and relieves Depression. It also moistens the Intestines and moves the stools. It strengthens Kidney Qi but disperses Congestion. When Damiana is combined with Saw Palmetto Berries, this combination is specific for prostate disease.

Radix Helionadis Dioicae is more commonly known as False Unicorn. It is a Blood-activating medicinal. It is Bitter and Warm and enters the Heart, Spleen, and Liver. It activates the Blood and transforms Stagnation, primarily in the Lower Burner. In addition, it clears and eliminates Damp Heat from the Lower *Jiao*.

Radix Collinsoniae Canadensis (Stone Root) is a Heat-clearing medicinal somewhat similar to Moutan. It is Acrid, Sour, and Cool. It enters the Liver, Pericardium, and Large Intestine Channels. It clears Ascending Liver Fire and clears and eliminates Damp Heat. Stone Root also strongly seeps Dampness and expels stones. In addition, it activates the Blood and disperses Stagnation. Stone Root has a special tropism for the Lower Burner and especially for the anal and perineal areas. In this formula, it assists False Unicorn in dispersing Stagnant Blood and Chaparral and Hydrangea in seeping Dampness and clearing Damp Heat.

Poria we have discussed above. In this formula, it addresses the Middle Burner as the typical source of Dampness. Thus this ingredient helps ensure that this formula addresses and regulates each of the three Burners in their role of transporting and transforming Liquids.

Rhizoma Dioscoreae Hypoglaucae is called in Chinese Bi Xie or Bie Xie and in Japanese Tokoro. It is a Damp-draining medicinal which is Bitter and Neutral. It enters the Liver, Stomach, and Bladder Channels. It separates Pure from Turbid and resolves Turbid Dampness in the Lower Burner. It also clears Damp Heat from the skin. In this formula, Tokoro assists Chaparral, Hydrangea, and Poria in draining Dampness and promoting urination. This ingredient is found in at least one Chinese empirical prescription for prostatic hypertrophy.

Semen Abutilonis Seu Malvae, or simply Abutilon, is another Damp-draining medicinal. Malva is a species of Ground Mallow. Malva Seeds are used to drain Dampness and promote urination in both Western and Chinese herbalism. They are used for *Re Lin, Xue Lin,* and *Shi Lin* as well as for *Shui Zhong* or edema. They moisten the Intestines and move the stool. Abutilon is Sweet and Cold and enters the three Bowels of the Lower Burner as well as the Liver.

As a whole, this formula rids Damp Heat from the Lower Burner, seeps Dampness and promotes urination, promotes the separation of Clear and Turbid in the Lower Burner, activates and courses the *Jue Yin* in the Lower Burner, activates and destagnates Blood in the Lower Burner, and tonifies the Kidneys and activates the Yang. Essence Chamber Tablets are especially useful for men between the ages of 40-60 in whom there is Dampness and Heat and some incipient decline of Kidney Qi but no clinical signs of Kidney Yin Deficiency.

Qian Lie Xian Wan (Prostate Gland Pills), a Chinese patent medicine, is somewhat similar in conception to Essence Chamber Tablets in that it also clears and eliminates Damp Heat. However, it focuses even more on activating the Blood and dispersing Stagnation. Although it is sold primarily for the remedial treatment of prostate hypertrophy and prostatitis, it can also be taken for 2-4 weeks at a time, once or twice a year by men over 40 as a preventive regime. Its ingredients are:

    Semen Vaccariae Segetalis
    Cortex Radicis Moutan
    Radix Paeoniae Rubrae
    Radix Astragali Seu Hedysari
    Herba Patriniae
    Radix Peucedani
    Radix Saussureae Seu Vladimiriae
    Caulis Akebiae Mutong
    Radix Glycyrrhizae

After 60 years of age and in persons with more obvious Yin Deficiency, Liu Wei Di Huang Wan (Rehmannia Six Flavors Pills) and/or Jie Jie Wan, called in Cantonese Kai Kit Wan (Dispelling Swelling Pills), may be used instead. The ingredients in Kai Kit Wan, aka Jie Jie Wan, are:

    Radix Rehmanniae Conquitae
    Radix Astragali Seu Hedysari
    Radix Codonopsis Pilosulae
    Fructus Ligustri Lucidi
    Semen Plantaginis
    Radix Achyranthis
    Radix Salviae Miltorrhizae
    Rhizoma Alismatis
    Semen Cuscutae
    Ootheca Mantidis

ORTHOMOLECULAR THERAPY

Zinc and Selenium are two very important minerals for the prevention of prostate problems and maintenance of prostate health. Zinc nourishes the Blood, strengthens the bones, brightens the eyes, and tonifies the *Jing* so as to support the Righteous in order to hold Evil in check. I advise men over 40 to take extra Zinc after ejaculation for a day or two. Zinc deficiency can be tested for by a Metagenics' product called Zinc Tally. It is a liquid Zinc preparation. If one does *not* taste a flat, metallic taste after holding a spoonful of Zinc Tally in their mouth for 30 seconds, they need extra Zinc. This test can be repeated over a period of several weeks to determine when no further supplemental Zinc is needed beyond normal maintenance levels.

Selenium benefits the Yin, restrains Floating Yang, settles and calms the Spirit, astringes the Essence, and enters the Liver and Kidney Channels. It also should be taken along with Zinc after ejaculation in men over 40.

Prostagen, a Metagenics' orthomolecular formula, can be taken preventively as well as remedially. Like Essence Chamber Tablets above and even along with Essence Chamber, it can be taken for several weeks at a time, 1-2 times per year. Those with known prostate problems can take this formula continuously. The ingredients of Prostagen are:

l-Glycine
l-Alanine
l-Glutamine
Raw Prostate Concentrate
Fructus Serenoae Serrulatae
Herba Solidaginis
Extractum Semenis Curcubitaceae

Vitamin E
Zinc Aspartate
Oleum Semenis Lini Usitatissimi

Glycine and Alanine are amino acids which nourish the substance of the prostate. Glutamic Acid is an amino acid which energizes the function of the prostate. Zinc benefits the *Jing* as does Vitamin E. Raw Prostate Concentrate benefits the prostate based on using the Organ or tissue to tonify that Organ or tissue. This is a principle of Chinese medicine dating to at least Zhang Zhong-qing of the Han, author of the *Jin Gui Yao Lue*.

Herba Solidaginis, aka Golden Rod, is Bitter, Astringent, and Cool and enters the Liver, Lungs, Bladder, and Triple Heater. It clears Heat, eliminates Dampness, and releases the Surface. It benefits Water and promotes urination. It is used for Wind Heat/ Wind Dampness upper respiratory tract catarrhs and Damp Heat *Lin*. It also treats borborygmus and flatulence due to Dampness in the Lower Burner impeding Small Intestine function.

Semen Curcubitaceae or Pumpkin Seeds are Sweet and Neutral and enter the Liver and Large Intestine. They expel Worms and alleviate pain as well as benefit postpartum Fluid metabolism, in which case they are indicated for edema of the hands and feet and insufficient lactation. The oil or concentrate is an empirical remedy for prostate problems.

Fructus Serenoae Serrulatae (Saw Palmetto Berries) has been described above under Essence Chamber Tablets.

Oleum Semenis Lini Usitatissimi or Flaxseed Oil, aka Linseed Oil, is also an empirical remedy for inhibiting tumor formation. It contains the essential fatty acid (EFA) Linoleic Acid. In TCM, it can be described as Sweet and Neutral. It nourishes and moistens the Intestines and moves the stool. It is a nourishing purgative. Flaxseed Oil probably enters the Liver, Lungs, and Large Intestine. It can be used for problems of the chest and breast, Gallbladder, constipation, and urination. Since it can be used as a poultice for Hot skin lesions the same as Semen Cannabis, Flaxseed Oil can also probably be said to clear Heat and promote the healing of sores.

For prostatitis and known or strongly suspected viral infection, up to several grams of Vitamin C can be taken daily to clear Heat and dissolve Toxins. The amount should always be less then that which causes loose stools or diarrhea so as not to weaken the Stomach/Spleen, the Root of Postnatal or Acquired Essence.

For older patients, typically over 60, who have a Dual Liver/Kidney Deficiency, Organic Germanium or Ge-132 is also a useful orthomolecular supplement for both the prevention and treatment of prostate problems. This mineral is a Yang tonic which nourishes the Liver Blood and tonifies both Kidney Yin and Yang. Therefore, it benefits the *Jing* Essence and promotes longevity. Like Epimedium, it also activates the Yang and harnesses Ascendant Liver Yang. It is specific for the treatment of the prostate. However, it should not be used by Yin Deficiency patients with Flaring of Deficiency Fire except sparingly and with care. Younger men over 40 may take Ge-132 after ejaculation along with Zinc and Selenium to more quickly replenish their *Jing*. If taken at too high a dose for too long a period by persons who are already relatively robust, Ge-132 can aggravate Evil Heat in the body. Therefore, although this medicinal is quite extraordinary, its use should be based on professional diagnosis. A very pure, high quality Organic Germanium is available from Bioenergy Nutrients of Boulder, CO. A typical preventive dose is 30 mg 2-3 times per day.

HOMEOPATHY & HOMOTOXICOLOGY

Homeopathy is another therapy which should be considered in dealing with chronic viral infections and the almost universal tendency of men to develop prostate cancer with age. Similar to our discussion of homeopathy above under CIN, there are modern, compound homotoxicological remedies to treat chronic viral infections. Apex Energetics markets a remedy called Post Virotox which is recommended for all chronic viral infections, such as EBV, HSV, CMV, etc. This is recommended to be taken with other of their formulas to aid the immune system. The other Apex formulas to be selected from include Immunosode, Immune Energy, Lymphotox, and Spleen Blood Activator. Using potentized resonance filters for determining biological age, efficacy, and tolerance, the most suitable combination of these remedies can be determined by Vega biokinesiology and/or electronic Vegatesting.

In addition, all men over 40 can take an Apex formula called Prostate Causal Chain in combination with Male Balance. Prostate Causal Chain is a compound formula specific for both the treatment and prevention of prostatitis, prostate hypertrophy, and prostate cancer. Male Balance helps balance the male endocrine system and regulates the hormones, and we have seen above the part male hormones play in the development of prostate cancer according to Western medicine.

Another homeopathic technique for the treatment of hidden viral infections revealed by electronic, biokinesiological, or DNA probe testing is the injection of homeopathic nosodes into acupuncture points. From the point of view of TCM, this is a species of *Shui Zhen* or Water Needle therapy. In Chinese Water Needle therapy, various liquid medicinals are injected into acupuncture points. These may be single herbal remedies made from Bupleurum, Dang Gui, Salvia, and Ginseng or compound herbal remedies such as Fu Fang Dang Gui Zhu She Ye (Compound Dang Gui Injectible). These may also be liquid vitamins, such as B_1 and B_{12}, or Western medicinals, such as Ringer's Solution and Procaine. In Europe, MDs practicing homeopathy often inject subcutaneously, intramuscularly, or even intravenously their liquid homeopathic medicinals.

Nosodes are homeopathic preparations made from sterilized disease products or from devitalized microbial cultures. Nosodes can be made from protozoa, bacteria, yeast, fungi, or viruses. Nosodes were first described in the homeopathic literature by Constantine Hering in the first part of the 19th Century. They are often very effective remedies when the Western pathogen can be determined. Patients testing positive for HPV or HSV II can be injected with the appropriate nosode during a course of treatment and then retested subsequently to see if the virus is still present in the body. Homeopaths believe that the use of nosode therapy in chronic diseases can help eliminate toxic substances from the body tissue which are then drained via the lymphatic system and excreted mainly by the kidneys. For men concerned with the health of their prostate, such injections can be given at Hui Yin (CV 1), Qu Gu (CV 2), and/or Heng Gu (Ki 11). Although I have only recently begun such treatments on men testing positive for HPV and HSV II, I believe such homeopathic *Shui Zhen* nosode therapy may prove effective. Injectible nosodes of HPV and HSV II are available from Arnica, Inc. of Santa Ana, CA in several different potencies.

Using either bioelectronic testing or biokinesiology with potentized resonance filters, practitioners can test to see which of the above combination of formulas, including Chinese herbal and orthomolecular regimes, gives the best therapeutic response and for how long they should be taken. This methodology is beyond the scope of this book. However, I do feel that homeopathic remedies may be one of our best therapies for negating Hidden Evils. Using the classical Chinese Four (Methods of) diagnosis, it is impossible to know whether a *Fu Wen Xie* has been eradicated from the body or not. Using these modern homeopathic *cum* electronic and/or biokinesiological methods, I think we can better gauge if and to what extent hidden viruses are causing an otherwise inexorable descent into disease. This is especially so with men who do not have the advantage of regular Pap smears.

ACUPUNCTURE

Although acupuncture can be an effective adjunctive therapy in the treatment of *Long Bi, Zhuo Lin, Qi Lin*, etc., in males over 40 years of age with no major complaints, I emphasize the sparing use of constitutional treatments. These treatments are based on Dr. Yoo's Three Constitutional Patterns. Although Dr. Yoo Tae-woo is primarily reknowned as the father of Korean Hand Acupuncture, I use his constitutional diagnosis co-ordinated with abdominal palpation and pulse to craft body acupuncture (*Ti Zhen*) treatments primarily utilizing the *Wu Shu Xue* or Five Transport Points.

By identifying the major Excess and Deficient Organs through the pulse and abdomen and rebalancing these every so often, ascension of the Clear and descension of the Turbid is regulated. This then results in the production of abundant Qi and Blood which can be converted into Acquired Essence and the elimination of Evil Accumulations such as Damp Heat and the Six Stagnations. In addition, I also often use *Qi Jing Ba Mai* or Eight Extraordinary Vessel treatments based on palpation, Manaka's Ion Pumping Chords, Zinc and Copper needles, and other state-of-the-art Japanese acupuncture techniques to achieve deep, constitutional rebalancing.

However, when treating constitutionally and asymptomatically,

I find that fewer treatments are more effective than frequent, repetitive ones. If the diagnosis and, therefore, the treatments are accurate and really touch the Root of the patient's dyscrasia, they will catalyze a long-lasting movement towards health. Immediately the treatment should result in sleep or very deep relaxation with REM (rapid eye movements), deepened breathing, minor involuntary twitching or movement, and/or possible tears. Similarly, the abdominal conformation should change by at least 50% and often there will be perceptible changes immediately in the pulse.

If treatment has catalyzed a deep movement towards health, it is sufficient to let this run its course for some time. Too frequent treatments rarely achieve any significant further benefit and typically eventually exhaust the therapeutic rapport between the patient and practitioner. This is called pushing the river. Rebalancing means reintegration and this is largely an unconscious process. Acupuncture treatments are best given only when this process has met a new snag requiring skilful intervention. This approach to acupuncture is like *Tai Ji* in which it is said that the force of a thousand pounds can be deflected by a few skillful ounces.

MASSAGE

In my practice I recommend asymptomatic, Root rebalancing acupuncture only infrequently -- for instance, at the change of seasons. Instead of weekly acupuncture, I highly recommend weekly or biweekly massage for health maintenance and disease prevention. I have described the TCM benefits of massage above under CIN. My only addition here is to once again recommend it enthusiastically.

SEX

A man is at greater risk for losing *Jing* Essence during sex than a woman. Although both men and women consume *Jing* by sex, men lose it in a way women do not. Therefore, sexual pacing is very important for men and especially after 40 years of age. On the one hand, too little sex can cause Stagnation of *Jing* which, in fact, is actually a Stagnation of Qi and Blood. On the other hand, too frequent ejaculation can cause exhaustion of *Jing* which then allows for flourishing of Hidden Warm Evils.

One Chinese formula for gauging safe frequency for ejaculation is to multiply one's age by 3, drop the zero or last digit, and divide by 2. The number that results is the number of days necessary to recuperate the *Jing* after an ejaculation. For instance, based on this system, a 40 year old man should ejaculate no oftener than every 6 days. Whereas, a 60 year old should only ejaculate once every 9 days.

A more conservative view is that held by Sun Si-miao of the Tang Dynasty. He felt that by one's 30s, men should ejaculate only once every couple of days. In their 40s, only once per week. In their 50s, only once every 2 weeks. At 60, once per month. And after that, not at all. Sun Si-miao lived to over 100.

These numbers should be adjusted for season of the year: spring and summer more, fall and winter less. They should also be adjusted for the patient's general health and vitality. Personally, I believe the main thing is being aware of the signs and symptoms of fatigue after ejaculation and being sensitive to how long it takes for these to recuperate before ejaculating again. Regimes like those described above are objective and, therefore, imprecise. Each man will vary all the time.

However, it is extremely important for men to know that, as they age, sexual pacing is a definite and important part of health maintainence and disease prevention. Here in the West, this is not widely known.

Beyond sexual pacing, condoms should be used with any new and especially casual sexual partners until their past venereal history is learned. If a woman has had cervical dysplasia which has been successfully treated, especially by the holistic methods described above, it may be assumed that her immune system has been provoked and is now competent to keep HPV in its latent and, therefore, non-transmissable form. Therefore, use of condoms with such partners may not be necessary. Men should definitely not have unprotected sex with partners of either sex who do have visible condylomatous lesions in the anogenital region.

CHAPTER TEN
THE REMEDIAL TCM TREATMENT OF PROSTATE PROBLEMS

My concern and focus in the previous chapter of this book has primarily been on how to prevent the occurrence of the epidemic of prostate problems I fear due to the wide spread of HSV and HPV amongst the Baby Boom generation. As mentioned at the beginning of the previous treatment section, I have only scant, personal clinical experience in treating prostate problems remedially. However, there are a few suggestions regarding their remedial treatment I would like to make.

The first is to begin treatment as early as possible. The warning signs are terminal dribbling, a weak stream or difficult urination, pinching pain on urination, turbid or cloudy urine, and pain in the perineal or prostate area. Those with a known history of herpes genitalia and genital warts should be especially diligent in treating and remedying these early warning signs. Acupuncture and Chinese herbal medicine prescribed and administered based on TCM *Bian Zheng* are effective for remedying the above complaints.

HERBAL THERAPY

Chinese herbal medicines for the remedial treatment of prostate problems can be administered either as high dosage decoctions for acute problems or as low dosage pills for chronic problems. As in all TCM Internal medicine or *Nei Ke*, the guiding formula is chosen based upon the TCM *Bian Zheng* diagnosis. There are a number of formulas suitable for the treatment of prostate problems depending upon the patient's personal Pattern (of Disharmony). Hong-yen Hsu, in "Chinese Herb Therapy for Benign Prostatic Hypertrophy" discusses relevant guiding prescriptions based on a Triple Heater classification of disease mechanism.[1] Based on literary research and disease mechanism theory I have made a number of additions to Dr. Hsu's suggestions for treating prostate problems and have also expanded his discussion of possible disease mechanisms under each Burner.

Upper Burner Disease Mechanisms

Even though the prostate is located in the Lower Burner, since Chinese medicine classifies prostate problems under urinary disturbances, and since TCM posits mechanisms accounting for urinary problems originating in all three Burners, it is possible to diagnose disease mechanisms for prostate problems due to pathological processes in the Upper Burner. In particular, the Lungs are responsible for controlling the Water Passageways or *Shui Dao* and for providing the motivating force for dispersing and descending Fluids downward. In addition, it is believed in TCM that Evil Heat may be passed from the Heart to its *Baio Li* paired Bowel, the Small Intestine, and thence to its *Tai Yang Liu Jing* pair, the Bladder. Therefore, Hsu gives two Upper Burner *Zheng* possibly accounting for certain individuals' prostate problems to which I have added three others.

1) Lung Heat

The signs and symptoms of Lung Heat obstructing the Lungs' dispersion and descension of body Fluids are dribbling, obstructed urination, a dry throat, irritability, thirst with a desire to drink, a slight cough, thick, yellow tongue fur, and a slippery, rapid pulse. Such Heat lingering in the Lungs is often due to Heat arising from the Liver and Stomach. In this case, there is typically some amount of concomitant Damp Heat in the Liver/Gallbladder. The guiding formula for Lung Heat urinary disturbance Dr. Hsu gives is Huang Jin Qing Fei Yin or Scutellaria Clear the Lungs Drink, aka Scutellaria & Gardenia Combination. I have not been able to find this formula in any English language source nor in any of my Chinese *Fang Ji Xue*. I believe Dr. Hsu may be referring to Qing Fei Yi Huo Wan (Clear the Lungs, Purge Fire Pills) since it includes Scutellaria and Gardenia and addresses the requisite treatment principles. Its ingredients are:

> Radix Scutellariae Baicalensis
> Fructus Gardeniae
> Radix Trichosanthis Kirlowii
> Radix Peucedani
> Radix Platycodi
> Rhizoma Anemarrhenae
> Radix Sophorae Flavescentis
> Rhizoma Rhei

Various Water-benefitting ingredients may be added to this guiding formula to make it more effective for treating Lung Heat urinary disturbance. These might include Semen Phaseoli Calcarati, Sclerotium Polypori Umbellati, Talc, Caulis Akebiae Mutong, etc.

2) Evil Water Wind Disturbing the Lungs

This Pattern is given by Ou-yang Yi in *A Handbook of Differential Diagnosis (&) Treatment, Vol. 1.*[2] It describes urinary difficulty due to a Wind Heat Invasion disturbing the Lungs' dispersion and descension. This then leads to an inability to dominate the Water Passageways and to move Fluids downward. Liu Yan-chi, in *The Essential Book of Traditional Chinese Medicine*, recommends Ma Huang Lian Qiao Chi Dou Tang (Ephedra, Forsythia, & Phaseolus Decoction) to treat this Pattern.[3] Its ingredients include:

> Herba Ephedrae
> Fructus Fosythiae
> Semen Phaseoli Calcarati
> Gypsum
> Rhizoma Imperatae
> Folium Perillae

If there is no hematuria, Imperata can be omitted and other Water-benefitting ingredients may be added as necessary. The difference between this Pattern and the preceding one is that Lung Heat is an Internal *Zheng*, while Wind Heat is an External Pattern. The signs and symptoms of Wind Heat invading the Lungs causing urinary disturbance are fear of chill, low back pain, facial edema and edema of the extremities, concentrated urine or hematuria, cough, shortness of breath, a pale but somewhat reddened tongue with a white coating (signifying a Superficial disease), and a floating, slippery pulse. In this case, a tendency towards chronic urinary problems may be suddenly exacerbated by a Superficial Wind Invasion, thus causing an acute urinary crisis. Ou-yang Yi gives another formula for essentially this same Pattern.[4] It is called Tong Guan Wan or Opening the Pass Pills. Its ingredients are:

> Herba Cum Radice Asari

>Folium Perillae
>Realgar
>Sclerotium Polypori Umbellati
>Spina Gleditschiae
>Rhizoma Alismatis
>Herba Menthae

3) Phlegm Dampness Obstructing the Lungs

Phlegm Dampness may accumulate in the Lungs again causing inability of the Lungs to disperse and descend. When this causes or contributes to urinary disturbances and difficulty, Ou-yang Yi calls this shutting above (causing) separation (from) below.[5] The basic signs and symptoms of this Pattern are cough with copious, wet Phlegm, stuffy chest, a white, greasy tongue coating, and a slippery, possibly forceless or even fine pulse. Ou-yang Yi suggests Er Chen Tang Jia Wei (Two Aged Decoction with Additions) for the treatment of urinary disturbances due to Phlegm accumulating in the Lungs.[6] Its ingredients are:

>Rhizoma Pinelliae Ternatae
>Sclerotium Poriae Cocoris
>Cortex Magnoliae Officinalis
>Pericarpium Citri Grandis
>Semen Pruni Armeniacae
>Semen Arecae
>Caulis Akebiae Mutong
>Fructus Citri Seu Ponciri
>Radix Glycyrrhizae

4) Dry Lungs, Fluid Injury

Due to Lung Yin Deficiency, the Lungs may also not be able to disperse and descend properly. Lung Yin Deficiency may be caused by a sudden, profuse loss of Liquids, such as through bleeding, diarrhea, vomiting, or excessive perspiration. However, it is more commonly met with during late summer and early autumn due to seasonal dryness and in arid areas. Living in Colorado, I see a fair amount of Lung Dryness problems and notice an increase of these in August and September when we can go two months or more without a drop of rain. The signs and symptoms of Lung Dryness causing urinary disturbance are a dry cough, adiaphoresis but often a sense of heat in the chest and upper back, and non-smooth urination. Ou-yang Yi does not give a named formula for this Pattern but recommends the following choice of herbs[7]:

>   Rhizoma Anemarrhenae
>   Radix Glehniae
>   Radix Asteris
>   Tuber Ophiopogonis
>   Rhizoma Polygonati Officinalis

In this case, it is assumed that urination will become normal as soon as the Lung Yin is tonified. Therefore, Ou-yang Yi has not included any Dampness-seeping ingredients which might only tend to aggravate this condition.

5) Heart Fire

As described above, Heart Fire, most often derived from mental and emotional stress, can be passed from Heart to Small Intestine and from Small Intestine to Bladder resulting in reddish and obstructed urination. The tongue is red, especially the tip, and most often there will be one or more sores or small ulcers at the tip. There is thirst, insomnia, possible palpitations, anxiety, and a rapid pulse. Dr. Hsu lists two guiding formulas for this type of urinary/prostate disorder, Dao Chi San and Qing Xin Lian Zi Yin.

Dao Chi San   (Conduct Red Powder, aka Rehmannia & Akebia Formula)

   Radix Rehmanniae
   Caulis Akebiae Mutong
   Herba Lophatheri Gracilis
   Radix Glycyrrhizae

Qing Xin Lian Zi Yin (Clear the Heart Lotus Seed Drink, aka Lotus Seed Combination)

   Semen Nelumbinis
   Radix Panacis Ginseng
   Radix Astragali Seu Hedysari
   Tuber Ophiopogonis
   Semen Plantaginis
   Cortex Radicis Lycii
   Sclerotium Poriae Cocoris
   Radix Scutellariae Baicalensis
   Radix Glycyrrhizae

This second formula is for Heat above and Deficiency below. It clears Heat from the Heart, Lungs, Stomach, and Liver at the same time as it tonifies both Pre and Postnatal Qi. In addition, it seeps Dampness from the Lower Burner.

Middle Burner Disease Mechanisms

Dr. Hsu only lists a single disease mechanism for urinary obstruction/prostate problems deriving from the Middle Burner. This is Damp Heat in the Middle Burner causing dysfunction in ascension and descension. Due to Dampness and Heat accumulating in the Middle obstructing the function of the Stomach/Spleen, Clear Qi cannot arise and Turbid Yin does not descend. This results in a mixed Excess/Deficiency

Pattern. The signs and symptoms of this Pattern are turbid and scanty urination, upper abdominal distention, a heavy feeling in the body, disinclination to talk, a pale tongue with a greasy coating, and a soft, forceless or fine pulse. The two guiding prescriptions Dr. Hsu lists for this Pattern are Bu Zhong Yi Qi Tang and Chun Ze Tang.

Bu Zhong Yi Qi Tang (Tonify the Middle and Benefit the Qi Decoction, aka Ginseng & Astragalus Combination)

  Radix Panacis Ginseng
  Radix Astragali Seu Hedyari
  Rhizoma Atractylodis Macrocephalae
  Radix Angelicae Sinensis
  Radix Bupleuri
  Rhizoma Cimicifugae
  Pericarpium Citri Reticulatae
  Fructus Zizyphi Jujubae
  Radix Glycyrrhizae
  Rhizoma Recens Zingiberis

Chun Ze Tang (Spring Pond Decoction, aka Ginseng & Hoelen 5 Combination)

  Radix Panacis Ginseng
  Radix Bupleuri
  Tuber Ophiopogonis
  Sclerotium Poriae Cocoris
  Sclerotium Polypori Umbellati
  Rhizoma Atractylodis Macrocephalae
  Rhizoma Alismatis
  Ramulus Cinnamomi

Lower Burner Disease Mechanisms

Dr. Hsu gives three basic Patterns (of Disharmony) of the Lower Burner describing urinary disturbances and, therefore, prostate problems. These are Damp Heat Accumulating in the Bladder, Damp Cold Obstruction and Stagnation of the Blood, and Deficiency Heat in the Lower Burner. To these I would add Obstructive Qi Stagnation.

1) Damp Heat Accumulating in the Bladder

We have discussed above the various mechanisms accounting for the accumulation of Damp Heat in the Bladder/Lower Burner. The textbook signs and symptoms of this Pattern are urinary obstruction, burning pain on urination, a hard, swollen lower abdomen resisting pressure, possible constipation, a greasy tongue coating at the root of the tongue, and a slippery, rapid pulse. However, the urine may be either dark yellow or red if there is predominant Heat or turbid and milky if there is predominant Dampness. The pulse may be deep and wiry in the *Chi* or Foot positions, the deepness signifying an Internal disease and the wiriness signifying the obstruction of the free-flow of Qi. In addition, if Dampness has compromised the Spleen's ability to *Sheng Hua* or create and transform the Qi and Blood, the pulse may be fine rather than obviously slippery. The two guiding prescriptions Dr. Hsu lists for Damp Heat Accumulating in the Bladder are Wu Lin San and Ba Zheng San.

Wu Lin San (5 *Lin* Powder, aka Gardenia & Hoelen Formula)

This formula is named for the Five *Lin* discussed above. However, based on an analysis of its ingredients, I would say that it is mostly for Damp Heat in the Lower Burner causing urinary disturbance due to Heat in the Liver complicated by

Liver Blood Deficiency. Its ingredients are:

> Radix Angelicae Sinensis
> Radix Paeoniae Albae
> Fructus Gardeniae
> Sclerotium Poriae Cocoris
> Radix Glycyrrhizae

Dang Gui and Peony nourish Liver Blood and relax the Liver, thus helping insure patency of the Qi. Gardenia clears Depressive and Damp Heat from the Liver. While Poria benefits Water and leads of Dampness. Licorice is added to detoxify and harmonize the formula. I believe that Licorice's harmonizing effect is mostly due to its benefitting the Heart. Since the Heart is the Ruler of the organism, strengthening that Organ has a systemic effect on the entire organism.

Ba Zheng San (8 Righteous Powder, aka Dianthus Formula)

This is a very commonly prescribed formula for urinary disturbances due to Damp Heat. It is composed almost entirely of Water-seeping medicinals. Its ingredients are:

> Herba Dianthi
> Semen Plantaginis
> Caulis Akebiae Mutong
> Fructus Gardeniae
> Medulla Junci Effusi
> Talc
> Herba Polygoni Avicularis
> Rhizoma Rhei
> Radix Glycyrrhizae

There are two other formulas for removing Damp Heat from the Lower Burner and facilitating urination that I would like to mention. These are Chou Xin Yin and Bie Xie Shen Shi

Tang.

Chou Xin Yin (Removing Firewood Brew)

The name of this formula is based on the mutual co-production of Dampness and Heat. It is Heat which stews the juices resulting in Damp Heat. This formula uses Heat-clearing medicinals to eliminate this Heat, thus eliminating one of the mechanisms producing Damp Heat in the Lower Burner. Use of these Heat-clearing medicinals is like pulling the wood out from under a pot boiling on top of a fire. The ingredients in this formula when modified to more effectively treat urinary disturbances include:

- Radix Scutellariae Baicalensis
- Fructus Gardeniae
- Cortex Phellodendri
- Caulis Akebiae Mutong
- Rhizoma Alismatis
- Rhizoma Dioscoreae Hypoglaucae
- Herba Dendrobii
- Fructus Immaturus Citri Seu Ponciri
- Excrementum Bombycis Mori
- Radix Glycyrrhizae

Bie Xie Shen Shi Tang (Tokoro Decoction for Permeating Dampness)

This formula is similar to the above in many regards. However, it includes Coix as one of its Water-seeping ingredients. If prostate problems are linked to HPV infection, this addition may turn out to be an important one since, as mentioned above, Coix possesses some specific anti-wart properties. The ingredients in this formula are:

- Rhizoma Dioscoreae Hypoglaucae

Cortex Phellodendri
Cortex Radicis Moutan
Talc
Semen Coicis Lachryma-jobi
Sclerotium Poriae Cocoris Rubrae
Rhizoma Alismatis
Medulla Tetrapanacis

2) Damp Cold Obstruction and Stagnation of the Blood

This Pattern is similar to Damp Cold Blood Stagnation dysmenorrhea. Its mechanism is that Dampness and Cold accumulating in the Lower Burner obstruct the flow of Qi and Blood eventually leading to Blood Stagnation. The signs an symptoms of this *Zheng* are urinary obstruction and dribbling and a distended lower abdomen which resists pressure but is benefitted by warmth. The tongue may be purple or ecchymotic. The pulse is typically deep at the *Chi* positions and wiry due to impatency. It may also be hesitant or, in more serious cases, irregular. Pain associated with this Pattern is usually pricking pain as opposed to burning pain. The two guiding formulas Dr. Hsu gives for this Pattern are Gui Zhi Fu Ling Wan and Hu Chang San.

Gui Zhi Fu Ling Wan   **(Cinnamon & Poria Pills, aka Cinnamon & Hoelen Formula)**

Ramulus Cinnamomi
Radix Paeoniae Rubrae
Cortex Radicis Moutan
Sclerotium Poriae Cocoris
Semen Pruni Persicae

Because this formula contains Cinnamom which is a Warm medicinal, it is listed here under Damp Cold Obstruction and

Stagnation. Most Chinese TCM practitioners say that Accumulation of Dampness and Cold are the two main reasons for Stagnant Blood in the Lower Burner. However, at least in the United States, this is not my experience. I find Dampness and Heat more often associated with Stagnation in the Lower Burner than Cold. If one analyzes the ingredients in the above formula, Red Peony and Moutan both clear Heat. In this case, Cinnamon is used in order to activate the Qi. Movement is Yang and Yang is Warm. Therefore, Qi and Blood flow when they are warm and warmth helps them flow better. In particular, Cinnamon benefits the Righteous Warmth of the Kidneys which supply the motivating power for the entire Lower Burner. If there is Cold causing Blood Stasis, Cinnamon does specifically treat this according to the logic of Chinese medicine. However, I believe it is preferable to simply title this category Stagnant Blood Obstructing the Lower Burner. If this category were so named, it would make more sense clinically and then, under this category would also be included formulas such as Teng Long Tang described in Chapter Six and Da Huang Mu Dan Pi Tang (Rhubarb and Moutan Decoction or Combination). The ingredients in this second formula are:

>Semen Benincasae Hispidae
>Cortex Radicis Moutan
>Semen Pruni Persicae
>Mirabilitum
>Rhizoma Rhei

Dr. Hsu does not give the ingredients for Hu Chang San in his article nor can I find this formula anywhere in the English or Chinese literature to which I have access.

3) Deficiency Heat in the Lower Burner

Although Dr. Hsu lists the above Pattern as a single mechanism for urinary obstruction, actually there are two different though related Patterns covered here. The first is Kidney Yin Deficiency accompanied by Deficiency Heat. The second is Kidney Yang Deficiency. As discussed above, in both instances there is Kidney Qi Deficiency causing lack of transportation and/or holding of the urine. In the case of Kidney Yin Deficiency, Deficiency Heat over-transforms the urine and so it tends to be scant and yellow. Whereas, in Kidney Yang Deficiency, lack of Heat causes insufficient transformation of Fluids resulting in excessive, clear, or pale urine. Typically as one ages, first one's Kidney Yin becomes Deficient and only later does one's Kidney Yang also becomes Deficient. When that happens one speaks of Kidney Yin and Yang Dual Deficiency. This is why Dr. Hsu only lists Deficiency Heat in his article since, in a sense, Kidney Yang Deficiency is only a further complication of Kidney Yin Deficiency in the elderly.

a) Kidney Yin Deficiency

The signs and symptoms of Kidney Yin Deficiency besides scant, yellow, frequent, and obstructed urination are nocturia, low back pain, fatigue, tinnitus, knee pain, dizziness, palpitations, and insomnia. The tongue is typically red with scant coating. It may also be apically fluted and/or cracked. If there are visible ulcers on the tongue, these tend to be mostly painless. The pulse may be fine and fast or may be fast, floating, and flooding. It is my experience that older patients with Kidney Yin Deficiency have this second pulse type which is not what most textbooks list. The guiding formulas for this type of urinary obstruction are Liu Wei Di Huang Wan and Chi Bai Di Huang Wan.

Liu Wei Di Huang Wan   (**Rehmannia 6 Flavors Pills**, aka **Rehmannia Six Formula**)

Radix Rehmanniae Conquitae

Radix Dioscoreae
Fructus Corni
Rhizoma Alismatis
Sclerotium Poriae Cocoris
Cortex Radicis Moutan

Zhi Bai Di Huang Wan (Anemarrhena & Phellodendron, Rehmannia Pills, aka Anemarrhena & Phellodendron Formula)

Radix Rehmanniae
Rhizoma Anemarrhenae
Cortex Phellodendri
Radix Dioscoreae
Fructus Corni
Sclerotium Poriae Cocoris
Rhizoma Alismatis
Cortex Radicis Moutan

The addition of Anemarrhena and Phellodendron to Liu Wei Di Huang Wan makes that formula more effective for treating Deficiency Heat effecting both the Upper and Lower Burners.

b) Dual Kidney Yin & Yang Deficiency

The signs and symptoms of simultaneous Yin and Yang Kidney Deficiency are fatigue, polyuria, nocturia, low back pain, cold extremities, chill in general, possible cockcrow diarrhea, incontinence, a pale tongue, and a sunken, weak, and possibly slow pulse. It is also possible in older patients to have Deficiency Heat manifesting in the Upper Burner with flushing-up signs and symptoms with Deficiency Cold symptoms manifesting or predominating in the Lower Burner. For this reason, the tongue and pulse signs are quite variable. Dr. Hsu lists two guiding formulas for treating Dual Kidney Yin & Yang

Deficiency urinary obstruction. These are Shen Qi Wan from the *Jin Gui Yao Lue* and Ba Wei Di Huang Wan. However, as far as I am concerned, these are one and the same formula.

Ba Wei Di Huang Wan (8 Flavors Rehmannia Pills, aka Rehmannia 8 Formula, aka Jin Gui Shen Qi Wan, aka Sexoton Pills)

Radix Rehmanniae Conquitae
Radix Dioscoreae
Fructus Corni
Sclerotium Poriae Cocoris
Rhizoma Alismatis
Cortex Radicis Moutan
Cortex Cinnamomi
Radix Praeparatus Aconiti Carmichaeli

Ou-yang Yi suggests that for the treatment of urinary disturbances due to Kidney Yin and Yang Deficiency, Semen Plantaginis and Semen Cuscutae should be added to the above formula to make it more effective for seeping Dampness.[8] There are also two other formulas I would like to mention for treating Kidney Yang Deficiency with Dampness and Turbidity obstructing urination. These are Bie Xie Fen Qing Yin Jia Wei and Chen Xiang San. The first is given by Yeung Him-che[9] and the second by Ou-yang Yi[10] for the treatment of urinary disturbances.

Bie Xie Fen Qing Yin (Tokoro Separate the Clear Drink)

This is one of two formulas of the same name. The other version of this formula will be described below. This formula was composed by Zhu Dan-xi in the Jin-Yuan Dynasty. Its ingredients when modified to make it more effective for the treatment of *Lin* diseases are:

  Rhizoma Dioscoreae Hypoglaucae
  Fructus Alpiniae Oxyphyllae
  Radix Linderae
  Rhizoma Acori Graminei
  Sclerotium Poriae Cocoris
  Radix Glycyrrhizae

This formula is indicated for the treatment of frequent urination with cloudy, "greasy" urine due to Deficiency Cold of the Lower Burner. In this case Kidney Yang is Deficient and thus there is insufficient Warmth to *Wen Hua* or transform Liquids in the Lower Burner. This results in the accumulation of Dampness below.

Chen Xiang San   (Aquilaria Powder)

This formula also treats Turbid Dampness in the Lower Burner due to Deficiency Cold and Kidney Yang's inability to properly transport and transform Fluids below. However, because this formula contains Semen Vaccariae, Peony, and Dang Gui, it also addresses the commonly encountered complication of Stagnant Blood as well. The ingredients in this formula are:

  Lignum Aquilariae Agallochae
  Talc
  Pericarpium Citri Reticulatac
  Radix Paeoniae Albae
  Radix Angelicae Sinensis
  Semen Vaccariae
  Herba Pyrrosiae
  Semen Abutilonis Seu Malvae
  Radix Praeparatus Glycyrrhizae

4) Obstructive Qi Stagnation

As discussed above under *Qi Lin*, Qi moves Water. It is the Liver which maintains patency of the Qi and is responsible especially for patency in the Lower Burner. If Liver Qi becomes congested, this may cause Stagnation and Accumulation of Liquids in the Lower Burner. Such Qi Stagnation is typically due to or is aggravated by emotional stress. Ou-yang Yi gives the signs and symptoms of Obstructive Qi Stagnation resulting in urinary difficulties as non-smooth urination, painful urination, a stuffy, distended lower abdomen, and a deep, wiry pulse. If there is pain, the pain usually precedes the flow of urine and as the urine is able to flow more smoothly, the pain diminishes or disappears. Ou-yang Yi recommends Qu Mai Tang in order to regulate the Qi and transport Liquids.[11]

Qu Mai Tang (Dianthus Decoction)

> Herba Dianthi
> Pericarpium Arecae
> Semen Pharbitidis
> Caulis Akebiae Mutong
> Rhizoma Belamcandae Chinensis
> Fructus Citri Seu Ponciri
> Rhizoma Et Radix Notopterygii
> Radix Angelicae Sinensis
> Radix Platycodi
> Rhizoma Corydalis Yanhusuo
> Rhizoma Coptidis
> Cortex Cinnamomi
> Rhizoma Rhei

This is a very interesting formula. Ou-yang Yi indicates it for the treatment of Liver Qi Stagnation dysuria, and it does contain Qi-regulating ingredients. However, it also deliberately addresses the Lungs as well through the inclusion of Belamcanda, Notopterygium, and Platycodon. In addition, it takes into account the Liver's relationship with the Large Intestine. The Liver and Lungs are the two Organs which control the Qi. The Lungs empower the movement of the Qi or supply it with its motivating force. They impel the Qi. The Liver maintains the patency of the Qi or its free-flow. In other words, the Liver allows the Qi to flow. The Liver accomplishes this through adjusting the lumena or openings of the Channels. The fact that many modern Western TCM theoreticians believe the Channels to be the fascial planes and the fact that classically the tissue associated with the Liver is the *Jin* helps explain further the Liver's role in maintaining the lumena of the Channels. In my experience, using the Lungs to control the Liver is a very effective way of re-establishing patency of Qi. In this particular case, since the Lungs also are one of the three Organs which control Fluids, this approach is even more insightful.

Besides these formulas based on relatively discrete or simple *Zheng*, there are a number of Chinese formulas for treating urinary disturbances which are based on the more complex or complicated Patterns described in the previous chapter. As mentioned above, prostate problems are often a combination of Dampness, Heat, Stagnant Qi, and Stagnant Blood all mutually entangled and obstructing each other. The following two formulas are representative of formulas designed to address this more complicated scenario.

Bie Xie Fen Qing Yin (Tokoro Separate the Clear Drink, *Yi-Xue Xin Wu* version)

This is the second of two formulas with the same name. The other of these two has been described above. According to Bensky and Barolet, this formula first appears in the *Yi Xue*

Xin Wu or *Medical Revelations*.¹² It clears Heat, eliminates Dampness, separates the Clear from the Turbid, but also disperses Stagnant Blood. It is indicated for terminal dribbling, one of the early warning signs of prostate problems. Its ingredients are:

>   Rhizoma Dioscoreae Hypoglaucae
>   Cortex Phellodendri
>   Rhizoma Acori Graminei
>   Sclerotium Poriae Cocoris
>   Rhizoma Atractylodis Macrocephalae
>   Radix Salviae Miltorrhizae
>   Semen Plantaginis

Hua Shi Tang (Talc Decoction)

This formula is for difficult urination with pain. In the preceding formula Salvia is for dispersing Stagnant Blood. In this formula, Vaccaria addresses that issue. Its ingredients are:

>   Talc
>   Semen Vaccariae
>   Semen Abutilonis Seu Malvae
>   Semen Plantaginis
>   Ramulus Cinnamomi
>   Radix Euphorbiae Kansui
>   Medulla Tetrapanacis
>   Folium Pyrrosiae

The above formulas may be used as appropriate during acute episodes in decoction in large doses with appropriate additions and subtractions based on the presenting signs and symptoms. For subacute, lingering urinary/prostate problems, it is usually better to use either pills or desiccated extracts. Many of the formulas listed above are available as desiccated extracts from Qualiherbs. There are also three Chinese herbal patent pills which are specifically for the treatment of prostate problems. All three have been mentioned above. They are Health Concerns' Essence Chamber Tablets, Jie Jie Wan (aka Kai Kit Wan), and Qian Lie Xian Wan. In addition, Liu Wei Di Huang Wan is available both as a Chinese patent pill and as Quiet Contemplative from K'an Herbs and Ba Wei Di Huang Wan is available as a Chinese patent and as Dynamic Warrior from K'an.

ORTHOMOLECULAR THERAPY

In addition to using Metagenics' Prostagen formula and taking extra Zinc and Selenium (available from Metagenics as E-400 Selenium), I recommend administering relatively high doses of Vitamin C during acute prostate problems. By high doses, I mean more than 1 g p.d. Several grams of Vitamin C can be taken up to the point that it causes loose stools. The amount should then be adjusted downward to the point where the stools are normal at the highest possible dose of C. Vitamin C's TCM description is that it clears Heat and dissolves Toxins. It is especially indicated for prostate problems due to Excess Heat and venereally-transmitted Evil Toxins.

ACUPUNCTURE

In terms of acupuncture, besides choosing points based on a combination of *Bian Zheng* and signs and symptoms, there are three Extra or non-meridian points which are useful in the treatment of urinary problems in general, including prostatitis, prostatic hypertrophy, and symptomatically in the treatment of prostate cancer. These are Hai Bao, Ma Kuai Shui, and Ma Jin Shui.

Hai Bao (Sea Seal) is located on the dorsum of the large toe in the center of the phalangeal joint at the medial side. It is indicated for *Shan Bing*. *Shan Bing* are diseases in men of the genital and inguinal region, including urinary and prostate problems. It is needled perpendicularly 0.1-0.3 *Cun* in depth. Needle the opposite side if the pathology is one-sided as in inguinal hernia.

Ma Kuai Shui (Horse Quick Water) is located 0.4 *Cun* below Quan Liao (SI 18). It is indicated for cystitis, polyuria, and *Lin* diseases. It is needled perpendicularly 0.1-0.3 *Cun* in depth. This point's name refers to being able to "pee like a horse" again after successful treatment.

Ma Jin Shui (Horse Gold Water) also refers to peeing like a horse. It is identical to Quan Liao (SI 18). It is indicated for kidney stones, nephritis, and lumbar sprain. It is needled perpendicularly 0.1-0.3 *Cun* in depth. Needling both Horse Quick Water and Horse Gold Water gets the best results in urinary problems. All three of these points are from Tung Ching-chang's Extra point protocols.[13]

PROSTATE MASSAGE

Intra-anal digital massage of the prostate can greatly help in cases of prostatitis and prostate hypertrophy. Urologists, GPs, and some massage therapists can perform this technique. Medical old-timers sometimes call this "milking the prostate". This is not a very elegant therapy, but it is extremely effective. TCM practitioners attempting to treat prostate problems should learn this technique. Essentially it consists of stroking the prostate forward and down. When prostate massage is coupled with acupuncture, Chinese herbs, and hydrotherapy, the results can be very satisfactory.

HYDROTHERAPY

Hydrotherapy is used in China, but it is a part of Chinese medicine which has yet to be incorporated into its American practice. In part, this is may be due to hydrotherapy's stemming from the folk tradition of Chinese medicine. However, hydrotherapy can be used very effectively for the treatment of both acute and chronic prostate problems.

For acute prostate problems, there are two basic treatments. If the condition is predominantly Hot, apply ice packs to the perineum or do cold water enemas in order to clear Heat. If the condition is predominantly due to Stagnant Qi and/or Blood, take hot sitz baths in order to activate the Qi and Blood.

For chronic prostate problems, one should vigorously spray the perineal area alternately with cold and then hot water. Cold water clears Heat and relieves inflammation. Hot water activates the Qi and Blood. Alternating the two both relieves inflammation and Stagnation. All three of these hydrotherapy treatments can be done daily at home by the patient himself, thus extending the scope of therapy and, therefore, its effectiveness. Men over 40 concerned about their prostates can also do this alternating cold then hot spray on their perineum on an occasional basis.

CONCLUSION

In this book I have suggested a relationship between at least two venereally transmitted viruses, HPV and HSV II, and cervical dysplasia/cervical cancer. I have then gone on to describe these viruses as *Fu Wen Xie* or Hidden Warm Evils from the point of view of TCM. And further, I have suggested that, due to the embryological similarity of the cervix and prostate, if these viruses cause cervical disease in women, it is likely that they might cause prostate disease in men. This line of reasoning is only just being investigated by Western researchers but I think it is quite likely.

Based on this hypothesis, I have presented treatment protocols for the remedial treatment of CIN in women and the prevention of prostate problems in men. These treatments have all been presented from the perspective of TCM theory but encompass therapies not usually associated with Chinese medicine in the West, such as orthomolecular therapy, homotoxicology, and hydrotherapy. I have expanded my treatment protocols for these and other related viral diseases beyond those that are traditionally Chinese in order to more comprehensively and effectively treat these problems. Busy clinicians interested solely in empirical results will probably find these treatments the most useful part of this book. However, for me, writing this book has mostly presented me with an opportunity for theoretical evolution.

Viral diseases are the single most important topic in medicine today. Western medicine has only recently geared up to meet this challenge. Likewise, Traditional Chinese Medicine will also have to grow and expand to adequately deal with all the ramifications of viral disease. In particular, as I hope I have shown, there needs to be renewed interest in *Wen Bing* theory and the subcategory of *Fu Wen Xie*. There also needs to be more attention paid to the whole category of *Bu Nei Bu Wai Yin* (Neither Internal Nor External Causes of disease) and especially to *Chong* or parasites (including yeast and protozoa), environmental toxins, iatrogenesis, geopathic, electromaganetic, and biorhythmic disturbances, and sexual injury (*Fang Lao*).

Hidden viruses, such as HPV, HSV, HIV, EBV, and CMV, all have a deleterious effect on the immune system. When the immune system is depressed, yeast, bacteria, and protozoa can proliferate and *vice versa*. Further, when yeast, for instance, proliferate in the bowels, healthy and pathologic commensal protozoa and bacteria lose their normal balance and dysbiosis takes place. Therefore, when treating viral infections, attention must be paid to the management of yeast, protozoa, and bacteria as well as to the direct treatment of viruses themselves. This can be accomplished in TCM under the rubric of *Bian Bing* diagnosis, e.g. candidiasis and amoebiasis, and Wu You-ke's statement, "One disease, one Qi." Also, regulation of the immune system via hormonal balance is also quite important. This further explains why regulation of the menses and treatment of menopathies is so important in the comprehensive treatment of CIN.

Attention to *Fu Wen Xie*, *Jun* (which specifically means yeast but in modern Chinese medicine generically refers to microbes), and *Chong* changes the complexion of TCM. Up till now, there has been an emphasis in American TCM on emotions, diet, and External pathogens in terms of pathogenic factors. And certainly these are significant pathogenic factors. But, by adding viruses, yeast, and protozoa, we not only create a more effective clinical medicine but one which combines the best of Western allopathic and naturopathic medicine with the best of Traditional Chinese Medicine.

It is not uncommon for an individual to be infected by more than one hidden virus at a time. Research indicates that such hidden viruses have a synergistic or cumulative effect on the organism. For instance, HIV infected women have a statistically significant greater incidence of HPV and cervical dysplasia than the HIV negative population.[1] This does not mean that HIV causes cervical dysplasia but that concurrent HIV infection allows for increased pathologic activity of other viruses, such as HPV and HSV, which might. This is definitely the case with HIV and HSV both I and II. HIV positives tends to manifest HSV infections as their condition worsens. This also goes for intestinal dysbiosis and parasitosis (chronic diarrhea) and candidiasis (oral thrush).

It is my opinion that it will be these hidden viral diseases which will catalyze the synthesis of TCM and Western medicine and the evolution of a universal New Medicine for the 21st Century. This book does nothing more than take some tentative steps in that direction. However, the journey of a thousand *Li* ...

APPENDIX I

Clinical Stages in Carcinoma of the Uterine Cerivx

Preinvasive Carcinoma

Stage O		Carcinoma in situ, intraepithelial carcinoma

Invasive Carcinoma

Stage I		Carcinoma strictly confined to the cervix
	Stage IA	Microinvasive carcinoma (early stromal invasion)
	Stage IB	All other cases of Stage I
Stage II		Carcinoma extends beyond the cervix but has extended to the pelvic wall. The carcinoma involves the vagina but not the lower 1/3.
	Stage IIA	No obvious parametrial involvement
	Stage IIB	Obvious parametrial involvement
Stage III		The carcinoma has extended to the pelvic wall. On rectal examination, there is no cancer-free space between the tumor and the pelvic wall. The tumor involves the lower 1/3 of the vagina.
	Stage IIIA	No extension to the pelvic wall

	Stage IIIB	Extension to the pelvic wall and/or hydronephrosis or non-functioning kidney
Stage IV		The carcinoma extends beyond the true pelvis or has clinically involved the mucosa of the bladder or rectum.
	Stage IVA	Spread of growth to adjacent organs
	Stage IVB	Spread to distant organs

APPENDIX II

Qin Bo-wei on the *Ming Men*

Qin Bo-wei was an important TCM author during the middle of this century. In *Qin Bo Wei Yi Wen Ji (The Collected Medical Writings of Qin Bo-wei)*, published by the Hunan Science & Technology Press in 1983, there is an essay on the *Ming Men*. In it, Qin Bo-wei describes the various inter-relationships between the *Ming Men* and the *Zang Fu*. Below is the chart Qin Bo-wei included in that essay. It summarizes these various inter-relationships.

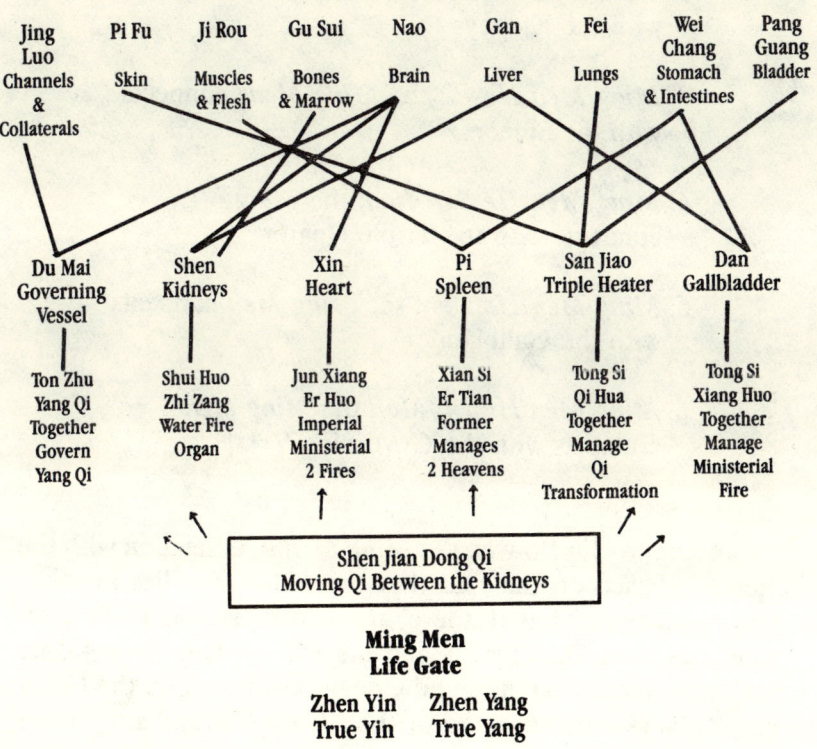

Below this chart, Qin Bo-wei then goes on to describe 6 inter-relationships between the *Ming Men* and other aspects of the human organism which he felt were important for TCM practitioners to understand. In each case, Dr. Qin uses the term *He*. This word means to unite. It is the same word which is used in describing the Lungs' relationship with the Large Intestine -- *Fei He Da Chang*; the Lungs are united with the Large Intestine. The following are a list of these 6 important *Ming Men* relationships:

1. *Ming Men He Xin*; the *Ming Men* connects with the Heart.

2. *Ming Men He Shen*; the *Ming Men* connects with the Kidneys.

3. *Ming Men He Pi*; the *Ming Men* connects with the Spleen.

4. *Ming Men He San Jiao*; the *Ming Men* connects with the Triple Heater.

5. *Ming Men He Dan*; the *Ming Men* connects with the Gallbladder.

6. *Ming Men He Du Mai*; the *Ming Men* connects with the Governing Vessel.

According to Qin Bo-wei, the *Ming Men*'s connection with the Heart is based on the fact that the *Ming Men* lies between both Kidneys and that there are Channels and Collaterals which connect the Kidneys and the Heart. Qin Bo-wei does not name these Channels and Collaterals; however, the Heart and Kidneys are connected by the *Chong Mai* and also by the

Bao Luo/Bao Mai. Although some authorities believe these are separate and discrete pathways, I think they are the same pathways given different names depending upon the body functions being described. In addition, Qin Bo-wei reiterates that the Heart is Imperial Fire, the *Ming Men* is Ministerial Fire, and that these two Fires are mutually interdependent and co-promoting. Specifically Qin Bo-wei says that *Ming Men Yang Qi* is connected with Heart Yang and that "once the *Ming Men Yang Qi* passes through the Heart Channel, it then possesses the ability to transmit the glow of the Essence Spirit through the entire body."

Qin Bo-wei explains the Kidneys' connection to the *Ming Men* as being both anatomical and functional. First he underscores the close anatomical position of the *Ming Men* nestled between the Kidneys. Then he goes on to discuss the fact that, according to the *Nei Jing*, "The Kidneys rule the bones and the bones generate Marrow," and that, "The brain is the Sea of Marrow." Because the Kidneys store *Jing* Essence and, therefore, control the containment and storage of the Root, "Thus it can be seen that the products of the Kidneys and bone Marrow, the activity of the brain, and the exuberance of the strength of reproduction all have an intimate relationship." Qin Bo-wei goes on to underscore the fact that the *Ming Men* plays an important role in all of these functions via the Kidneys.

As for the Spleen's connection to the *Ming Men,* Qin Bo-wei discusses this in relationship to Former (*Xian*) and Latter (*Hou*) Heaven (*Tian*) or Pre and Postnatal energies. As Qin Bo-wei says, "The generation and transformation of Latter Heaven is necessarily dependent upon the warmth and nourishment of Former Heaven's Life Fire." Interestingly, Qin Bo-wei then says that Kidney Yin or the "True Yin of Former Heaven" must necessarily be continuously supplied to Latter Heaven. This means that *Jing* Essence is continuously expended in the creation postnatally of Qi and Blood. However, excess Qi and Blood are transformed into Acquired Essence to be stored in the Kidney, there to bolster Prenatal Essence. Qin Bo-wei first quotes Xu Shu-wei: "Fortify the Spleen if not fortify the Kidneys." Then he quotes Li Dong-yuan who said, "Fortify the Kidneys if not the Spleen." Both these quotes underscore the Spleen and Kidneys' close, mutual relationship which, as I see it, involves not only Pre and Postnatal Yang but Pre and Postnatal Yin as well. This describes both the inseparability of Yin and Yang and Former and Latter Heavens.

Qin Bo-wei's discussion of the *Ming Men*'s connection with the Triple Heater is likewise based on classical Chinese Source theory. Qin Bo-wei says:

> *Ming Men* is the Source of the Triple Heater. Tang Yong-chuan referred to it as the burning source (*Jiao Yuan*) and the *Nei Jing* says that, "(The Triple Heater) belongs to the Kidneys and upwardly connects the Kidneys with the Lungs." The *Ming Men Yang Qi* warms the interstitial striae and via the Triple Heater envelops the entire body. *Ying Qi* issues from the Middle Burner and *Wei Qi* issues from the Lower Burner. This too (i.e. *Ying* and *Wei*) passes through the Triple Heater (where it) is generated and transformed.

As for the *Ming Men*'s connection with the Gallbladder, Qin Bo-wei says that both the *Ming Men* and the Gallbladder are Ministerial Fire. Life Fire, short for *Ming Men Zhi Huo*, the Fire of the Gate of Life, warms and nourishes Gallbladder Fire. It is the warmth of the Gallbladder which is responsible for the spring-like Qi of the Liver being patent or free-flowing. This line is pregnant with meaning, at least when written in

Chinese. The right hand side of the character for Gallbladder (*Dan*) depicts the sun rising over the horizon. The implication is that Gallbladder/Ministerial Fire warms the Liver in the same way that the sun warms the earth to make things flow and grow in the spring. "It is for this reason that our ancestors considered the Gallbladder the Righteous Center and also held that all the other 11 *Zang* are dependent on it."

This is a very interesting series of statements since nowhere else in the English language literature am I aware of a discussion of the actual mechanics of the Liver's maintaining patency of the Qi. In TCM, warmth is believed to promote flow just as in nature a lack of warmth causes freezing and lack of flow. It is the warmth of the Gallbladder which promotes the patency of Liver Qi. This helps to explain why, when Liver Qi becomes impatent, it so quickly transforms into Evil Heat. This line also underscores the fact that if the Liver is impatent, Qi and Blood do not flourish and expand in the same way that unwarmed earth is not the medium for the exuberant growth of spring.

Qin Bo-wei's discussion of the connection between the *Ming Men* and the Governing Vessel evidences the fact that Chinese medicine has two different theories concerning mind and consciousness which it has never been able to entirely unify. He begins by saying that the *Ming Men Yang Qi* is transmitted to the Twelve Regular Channels by the Governing Vessel. He then goes on to link the Governing Vessel to the Kidneys below and the brain above thus reiterating again the *Ming Men*'s connection with the Kidneys and the brain. This theory derives from Daoist inner alchemy and yogic practices. It is the Chinese version of *Kundalini* theory. Contemporary Chinese practitioners of TCM, it seems to me, always like to emphasize this theory since it is analogous to Western anatomy and physiology. Modern Chinese practitioners of TCM are not entirely comfortable with the idea that consciousness resides in the Heart. Qin Bo-wei indicates this dual theory in his chart with its connections between the *Ming Men, Du Mai*, brain and Heart.

Be that as it may, these inter-relationships between the *Ming Men* and the rest of the organism must be understood if one is to gain a deeper appreciation of the role of Heat as a pathogen and the various disease mechanisms which are derived from the above theories. With such an understanding one can follow the evolution and progression of complicated diseases. Without it, one is left with the static snapshots TCM calls *Zheng* or Patterns (of disharmony).

APPENDIX III

Naturopathic Treatment Schedule For Escarotic Therapy In CIN

Based on clinical results at the
Portland Naturopathic Clinic
Compiled by Toni Hudson, ND

Mild Dysplasia, CIN 1 without Condyloma

Topical treatment spans 4 weeks.

Week 1	Nightly Vitamin A emulsion on the end of a tampon inserted into the vagina
Week 2	Nightly vaginal suppository comprised of: Myrrha, Radix Echinacae Angustifoliae, Lichenificatio Usneae, Radix Hydrastis Canadensis, Radix Altheae Officinalis, Radix Geranii Maculati, Herba Achilleae Millefolii
Week 3	Repeat week 1's regime
Week 4	Repeat week 2's regime
Weeks 1-4	Use an escarotic Vag Pack 1 time per week for 12 hours followed by a dilute apple cider vinegar douche. This naturopathic escarotic Vag Pack is comprised of: Anhydrous $MgSO_4$, Glycine, Hydrastis Tincture, Tea Tree Oil, Thuja Oil, Bitter Orange Oil, Ferric Sulphate,

Ferrous Sulphate, and Aluminum Sulphate wrapped in cotton gauze and inserted into the vagina against the cervix. It is available from the Eclectic Institute of Portland, OR.

Repeat Pap 1 month after last escarotic treatment during which time only Vitamin A is used topically.

Mild Dysplasia, CIN 1 with Condyloma

Treat as above but for 8 weeks instead of 4. After discontinuing escarosis, use Vitamin A emulsions and Slippery Elm suppositories, alternating weekly for 1 month before getting a repeat Pap.

Moderate Dyspalsia, CIN 2 without Condyloma

Treat as above for 6 weeks with escarosis 1 time per week. Again wait 1 month before repeat Pap.

Moderate Dysplasia, CIN 2 with Condyloma

Treat the same as for CIN 1 with condyloma.

Severe Dysplasia & CIS, CIN 3 with or without Condyloma

Topical treatment spans 5 weeks. Escarotic therapy is done 2 times per week for a total of 10 treatments. Again wait 1 month using weekly alternating Vitamin A emulsion and Slippery Elm suppositories before repeat Pap.

APPENDIX IV

Dietary Considerations For Candidiasis

A. Some authorities suggest a high protein, low carbohydrate diet. One problem associated with this diet is the fact that a high protein diet is typically also high fat. High fat diets are associated with increased risk of cancer, cardiovascular disease, and a host of other problems. They are also well known to be immunosuppressive. With this in mind, I believe the best aproach is a modified Pritikin or Macrobiotic diet. That is a diet deriving about 60% of its calories from complex carbohydrates, 20% from protein, and 20% from fat. The key to this diet is that the carbohydrates should be supplied in their complex form. This means:

100% whole grain, non-instant wheat, rice, millet, buckwheat, or corn cereals

All fresh, lightly cooked vegetables with skins on, alone or in combination with any other allowable foods, such as stews, soups, and casseroles served warm

Fish, shell fish, white meat turkey without the skin, very lean red meats, baked, broiled, or stewed, not fried; use water-packed tuna, sardines, salmon, etc.

Whole eggs poached or soft boiled in moderate amounts, 3-5 per week

Kidney, pinto, navy, chick, soy, black, and garbanzo beans, and all peas in soups, stews, casseroles with any other allowable foods served warm

Water, especially spring water and herb teas

Limited amounts of fruit with fruit choices coming from those fruits which tend not to mould, i.e. apples, pears, bananas

B. Eliminate yeast and fungi containing foods such as:

Brewer's yeast, baker's yeast, and all foods whose preparation obviously depends upon yeast and fermentation, such as breads, rolls, hamburger buns, cake, cake mixes, coffee cakes, cookies, crackers, pretzels, most pastries, and most enriched flour products

Edible fungi, such as all types of mushrooms, truffles, morels

Mold-containing foods, such as all cheeses, including Swiss, cream, and cottage cheese, Velveeta, macaroni and cheese, and cheese containing snacks, buttermilk, sour cream, and sour milk products

Peanuts and peanut-containing products

Condiments, sauces, all types of vinegar (apple, wine, distilled), and vinegar-containing foods, processed and smoked meats, and malt products (cereals, candy, malted milk drinks)

Alcoholic beverages, such as wine, beer, rum, vodka, brandy, gin, whiskey, and other fermented liqours and liquers

Other fermented beverages, such as cider and root beer

C. Eliminate all simple and refind sugars such as:

Sucrose, fructose, maltose, lactose, glucose, and other

monosaccharides

Honey, molasses, maple syrup, maple sugar, date sugar, barley malt

Dried and candied fruits, such as raisins, apricots, dates, prunes, figs, and pineapple

Melons, including honeydew and cantaloupe

Fruit juices, either canned, bottled, or frozen, including orange, grape, apple, tomato, and pineapple juices

Packaged and processed foods that are either canned, bottled, boxed, or packed which usually contain yeast or refined sugar products

Soft drinks sweetened with refined sugars

APPENDIX V

Pygeum Africanum

As we were going to press with this book, I found the following information on an African herbal medicinal called Pygeum and its effects on benign prostatic hypertrophy (BPH). This information was contained in an article by Daniel B. Mowrey, Ph.D, entitled "Pygeum for the Treatment of Benign Prostatic Hypertrophy" appearing in the July/August 1990 issue of *Health World* (p. 16-20). Although I have no personal experience using this herb in the treatment of BPH, because this medicinal seems to be quite effective in treating this disorder, I have chosen to include this last minute appendix devoted to it.

Pygeum Africanum, aka Prunus Africana, is a large evergreen tree native to high plateaus in southern Africa. Its use is mentioned in botanical texts from the second half of the 18th Century. It seems that from its earliest medicinal use, Pygeum has demonstrated an ameliorating effect on BPH. Dr. Mowrey says that decades of research have now been done on Pygeum confirming both Pygeum's efficacy on BPH and its Western pharmacological lines of action.

According to Dr. Mowrey, Pygeum acts as an anti-inflammatory due to its plant sterols which inhibit prostaglandin biosynthesis. By reducing inflammation, these sterols also indirectly reduce the *tumor* or swelling associated with inflammation. This results in shrinkage of an inflamed prostate. Secondly, the pentacyclic triterpenoids in Pygeum inhibit the enzymes found in the initial phases of inflammation. And third, Pygeum's linear alcohols and ferulic esters inhibit the absorption and metabolism of cholesterol. Dr. Mowrey mentions that cholesterol has been suspected as being the root cause of BPH for some time.

The first two lines of action of this herb continue to suggest to me the possibility of a viral etiology in prostate problems. Pygeum helps shrink enlarged prostates by relieving inflammation. But what causes this inflammation in the first place? Even the third line of action, the inhibition of the absorption and metabolism of cholesterol, may still have something to do with viruses.

Cholesterol is manufactured in the liver. It is not just something we get from certain foods which we eat. As Drs. Stoff and Pellegrino explain in *Chronic Fatigue Syndrome, The Hidden Epidemic* (Harper & Row, NY, 1990, p. 98-9), long-term stress (and sugar consumption) causes the adrenals to secrete cortisone and chronically elevated cortisone levels may suppress the immune system. Cortisone also causes the liver to gear up for long-term endurance. It increases its storage of glycogen and its manufacture and release of cholesterol. Therefore, elevated serum cholesterol is a often a symptom of long-term stress, a compromised immune system, and consequently persistent viral infection.

Because decreasing the concentration of cholesterol in cell membranes makes it harder for lipid-coated viruses, including HIV, EBV, CMV, other herpes viruses, and hepatitis B, to attach themselves to receptor sites on these membranes, Stoff and Pellegrino recommend a low cholesterol diet for remedying and preventing persistent viral infections. It is entirely possible for Pygeum to reduce cholesterol and benefit the prostate without ruling out a viral co-factor in BPH.

Pygeum Africanum Extract with 13% guaranteed sterols is marketed in capsule form by Solaray of Ogden, UT. Its use, both preventively and remedially, is perhaps especially indicated in men with high serum cholesterol.

APPENDIX VI

Distributors of Medicinals Described in Text

Arnica, Inc.
144 E. Garry Ave.
Santa Ana, CA 92707
(714) 545-8203

Eagle Marketing Inc.
425 Calle Primera, Suite 102
San Ysidro, CA 92073
1-800-359-3245

Eclectic Institute, Inc.
11231 S.E. Market St.
Portland, OR 97216
1-800-332-HERB

Health Concerns
2236 Mariner Square Drive #103
Alameda, CA 94501
1-800-233-9355

K'an Herbs
2425 Porter St., Suite 18
Soquel, CA 95073
1-800-543-5233

Mayway Trading Co.
622 Broadway
San Francisco, CA 94133
(415) 788-3646

Metagenics International
971 Calle Negocia
San Clemente, CA 92629
1-800-692-9400
(call for phone # of regional distributor)

Qualiherbs
13340 E. Firestone Blvd., Suite N
Santa Fe Springs, CA 90670
1-800-533-5907

Scientific Botanicals
P.O. Box 31131
Seattle, WA 91203
(818) 243-5336

Seven Forests
Distributed by Health Concerns
(see above)

Solaray
2815 Industrial Dr.
Ogden, UT 84401

Yerba Prima Botanicals
P.O. Box 2569
Oakland, CA 94614
1-800-421-9972

ENDNOTES
Endnotes to Chapter One

1   Barber, Hugh K., *Manual of Gynecologic Oncology, Second Edition*, J.B. Lippincott Co., Philadelphia, 1989, p. 219

2   Karp, Shelley et al., *Cancer in Colorado Women 1979-1985, Prevention, Incidence, Survival, and Mortality*, American Cancer Society, Denver, undated, p. 31

3   Barber, op.cit., p. 217

4   Ferenczy, Alex, M., M.D., in "HPV DNA: Quicker Ways to Discern Viral Types", a symposium appearing in *Contemporary OB/GYN*, April, 1989, p. 2

5   Reid, Richard, M.D., Ibid., p. 5

6   Karp, op.cit., p. 33

7   Ferenczy, Alex, M.D. et al., "Latent Papillomavirus and Recurring Genital Warts," *The New England Journal of Medicine*, September 26, 1985, Vol 313, No. 13, p. 784

8   Barber, op. cit., p. 205

9   Nelson, James, H., Jr., M.D. et al., "Dysplasia, Carcinoma In Situ, and Early Invasive Cervical Carcinoma," *Ca-A Cancer Journal for Clinicians*, American Cancer Society, Nov./Dec. 1984, Vol 34, No. 6, p. 320

10   Barber, op.cit., p. 205

11   *The Merck Manual of Diagnosis and Therapy*, 15th Edition, Robert Berkow, ed., Merck, Sharp, & Dohme Research Laboratory, Rahway, NJ, 1989, p. 1726

12   Muñoz, N. et al., "Does Human Papillomavirus Cause

Cerivcal Cancer? The State of the Epidemiological Evidence," *The British Journal of Cancer*, Vol. 57, p. 1

13   Nelson, op.cit., p. 313

14   Barber, op.cit., p. 216

15   Ibid., p. 216

16   Nelson, op.cit., p. 313

17   Muñoz, op.cit., p. 1

18   Ferenczy, "Latent Papillomavirus . . .", op.cit., p. 786

19   Larsen, Peter Mose *et al.*, "Future Trends In Cervical Cancer," *Cancer Letters*, Elsevier Scientific Publishers Ireland, Ltd., No. 41, 1988, p. 126

20   Ibid., p. 125

21   Koutsky, Laura A. *et al.*, "Epidemiology of Genital Human Papillomavirus Infection," *Epidemiological Reviews*, The Johns Hopkins Univeristy School of Hygiene & Public Health, Vol. 10, 1988, p. 151

22   Lancaster, Wayne D. & Jenson, A. Bennett, "Natural History of Human Papillomavirus Infection of the Anogenital Tract," *Cancer and Metastasis Reviews*, Martinus Nijhoff Publishers, Boston, Vol. 6, 1987, p. 657

23   Sixby, John W. *et al.*, "A Second Site for Epstein Barr Virus Shedding: The Uterine Cervix," *The Lancet*, November 15, 1986

24   Bevan, I.S. *et al.*, letter to editor, *The Lancet*, April 22, 1989

25   Javier, R.T. *et al.*, letter to editor, *Science*, Vol. 234, p. 746

26 Pizzorno, Joseph E. & Murray, Michael T., *A Textbook of Natural Medicine*, Vol. 1, John Bastyr College Publications, Seattle, 1987, VI: Cer Dys

27 Wilie-Rosett, J.A. et al., "Influence of Vitamin A on Cervical Dysplasia and Carcinoma In Situ," *Nutrition and Cancer*, Vol. 6, No. 1, 1984, p. 49-57

28 Romney, S.L. et al., "Plasma Vitamin C and Uterine Cervical Dysplasia," *American Journal of Obstetrics & Gynecology*, Vol. 151, No. 7, 1985, p. 976-980

29 Butterworth, C.E. et al., "Improvement in Cervical Dysplasia Associated with Folic Acid Therapy in Users of Oral Contraceptives," *American Journal of Clinical Nutrition*, No. 35, 1982, p. 73-82

30 Ramaswamy, P. & Natarajan, R., "Vitamin B_6 Status in Patients with Cancer of the Uterine Cervix," *Nutrition and Cancer*, Vol. 6, 1984, p. 176-180

31 Prasad, K. ed., *Vitamins, Nutrition, and Cancer*, Karger, NY, 1984

32 Dawson, E. et al., "Serum Vitamin and Selenium Changes in Cervical Dysplasia," *Fed. Proc.*, Vol. 43, No. 612, 1984

33 Brandes, J. et al., "The Diagnostic Value of Serum Copper/Zinc RAtio in Gynecological Tumors," *Octa Ob/Gyn Scandinavia*, Vol. 62, 1983, p. 226-229

34 Barnet, T.J. et al., "Genital Warts -- A Venereal Disease," *Journal of the American Medical Association*, Vol. 154, 1954, p. 333-334

35 Koutsky, op.cit., p. 142

36 Lancaster & Jenson, op.cit., p. 660

37   Ibid., p. 660

38   Ibid., p. 655

39   Carson, L.F. *et al.*, "Human Genital Papilloma Infection: An Evaluation of Immunologic Competence in the Genital Neoplasia-Papilloma Syndrome," *American Journal of Obstetrics & Gynecology*, No. 155, 1986, p. 784-789

40   Lancaster & Jenson, op.cit., p. 655

41   Lipshultz, Larry I., M.D., "Condyloma," zeroxed handout, Baylor College of Medicine, Department of Urology, P. 2

42   Ibid., p. 1

43   Elman, M. Ian, "Other Sexual Diseases Overshadowed by AIDS," *Colorado Daily*, Feb. 6, 1990, p. 5

44   Koutsky, op.cit., p. 140
45   Ferenczy, in "HPV DNA ...," op.cit., p. 1-2

46   Becker, Thomas M., M.D., Ibid., p. 4

47   Ferenczy, Ibid., p. 7

48   Townsend, Duane E., M.D., Ibid., p. 11

49   Ferenczy, Ibid., p. 11

50   Reid, Richard M., M.D., Ibid., p. 7

51   Hatch, Kenneth D., *Handbook of Colposcopy: Diagnosis and Treatment of Lower Genital Tract Neoplasia and HPV Infections*, Little, Brown, and Co., Boston, 1989, p. 53

52   Ibid., p. 55

53   The term vicariation in relationship to the course of disease

is taken from Dr. Hans-Heinrich Reckeweg, the founder of homotoxicology. For further information on this theory see: Reckeweg, Hans-Heinrich, *Homotoxicology: Illness and Healing Through Auto-homotoxic Therapy*, Menaco Publishing Co., Albuquerque, NM, 1989

54 Lipshultz, op.cit., p.3

55 Hatch, op.cit., p. 64

56 Ibid., p. 73

57 Koutsky, op.cit., p. 151

58 *The Merck Manual*, op.cit., p. 250

Endnotes to Chapter Two

1 Modern TCM texts repeat over and over again that the foundation of TCM methodology is diagnosis by *Bian Zheng*. This term, *Bian Zheng*, is of relatively recent origin. Its state endorsed usage stems from the fact that this term is also part of the name of a communist doctrine: dialectical materialism (*Zi Jen Bian Zheng Fa*). According to Paul U. Unschuld (*Medicine In China, A History of Ideas*, University of California Press, Berkeley, 1985, p. 248), this term was transferred to the medical sphere based on articles which appeared in a journal entitled *The Dialectic of Nature* published in shanghai from 1973-1976.

2 Zhang Dai-zhao, *The Treatment of Cancer by Integrated Chinese-Western Medicine*, trans. by Zhang Ting-liang & Bob Flaws, Blue Poppy Press, Boulder, CO, 1989

3 Hsu, Hong-yen, *Treating Cancer with Chinese Herbs*, OHAI, Los Angeles, 1982, p. 73-75

4   Zhang, op.cit., p. 83-86

5   Jia Kun, *The Prevention and Treatment of Carcinoma in Traditional Chinese Medicine*, The Commerical Press, Hong Kong, 1985, p. 79

6   This is in contradistinction to what most Chinese TCM practitioners say. Most Chinese doctors say that Stagnant Blood due to Obstruction by Cold and Dampness is the leading cause of *Shao Fu Tong* and *Tong Jing*. This discrepancy may be due to either different etiologies and constitutions between Chinese and Americans or a different interpretation of certain key TCM prescriptions, such as Wen Jing Tang. Many prescriptions effective for the treatment of dysmenorrhea include Ramulus Cinnamomi. Based on strict modern TCM heteropathic methodology, one can only prescribe Cinnamon if the TCM diagnosis includes Cold. However, Cinnamon can also be used to dissipate Internal Heat by diaphoresis and to activate the flow of Qi and Blood without there necessarily being the presence of pathologic Cold.

7   Jia Kun, op. cit., p. 77

8   Jin Zi-jiu, "Jin Zi-jiu's Medical Contemplations," trans. by Michael Helme, *Timing and the Times*, Blue Poppy Press, Boulder, CO, 1986, p. 128

9   *Revised Outline of Traditional Chinese Medicine,* trans. by Nathan Sivin, excerpted and appearing in *Traditional Medicine in Contemporary China*, Ann Arbor, 1987, p. 381

10 *Nei Jing Su Wen*, quoted by Wu Bo-ping & Lu Shou-kang, "AIDS, A Preliminary Study of Symptom-Sign Complexes and Treatment," trans. by C.S. Cheung, *Journal of the American College of Traditional Chinese Medicine*, #2, 1987, p. 45

11 Liu Yan-chi, *The Essential Book of Traditional Chinese*

Medicine, Vol I, Columbia University Press, NY, 1988, p. 279

12   Wu & Lu, op.cit., p. 45

13   Ibid., p. 45

14   Jia Kun, op.cit., p. 79

15   Flaws, Bob, letter to the editor, *Dialogues*, Denver, Vol 2, #3, May, 1988, p. 16-18

16   Unschuld, Paul, U., op.cit.

17   Lu Gwei-djen & Needham, Joseph, *Celestial Lancets, A History and Rationale of Acupuncture and Moxa*, Cambridge University Press, Cambridge, 1980

18   Sivin, Nathan, *Traditional Chinese Medicine in Contemporary China*, Center for Chinese Studies, University of Michigan, Ann Arbor, 1987, p. 47

19   Koutsky, op.cit., p. 141

20   Zhang, op.cit., p. 84-86

21   Hsu, op.cit., p. 75

22   Flaws, Bob, *Sticking to the Point, A Rational Methodology for the Step by Step Formulation & Administration of an Acupuncture Treatment*, Blue Poppy Press, Boulder, CO, 1990

Endnotes to Chapter Three

1   Flaws, Bob & Wolfe, Honora Lee, *Prince Wen Hui's Cook, Chinese Dietary Therapy*, Paradigm Publications, Brookline,

MA, 1983

2 Flaws, Bob, *Nine Ounces, A Nine Part Program for the Prevention of AIDS in HIV Positive Persons,* Blue Poppy Press, Boulder, CO, 1989

3 Hlavaty, Vaclav, M.D., "Preface," *Children of Your Own: The Mojzis Method* by Ludmila Mojzis, Richmond Bay Publishers, Boulder, CO, 1989, p. vi

4 Song Guang-ji & Yu Xiao-zhen, *A Handbook of Traditional Chinese Gynecology,* trans. by Zhang Ting-liang & Bob Flaws, Blue Poppy Press, Boulder, CO, 1987

5 Cheung, C.S., *On Prescription,* Vol. 2, Harmonious Sunshine Cultural Center, S.F., 1988, p. 44-76

6 Hsu Hong-yen, *Treating Cancer with Chinese Herbs,* op.cit., p. 76-77

7 Wiseman, Nigel & Ellis, Andrew, *Fundamentals of Chinese Medicine,* Paradigm Publications, Brookline, MA, 1985, p. 356

8 Liu, op.cit., p. 280

9 Dharmananda, Subhuti, *Prescriptions on Silk and Paper,* Institute for Traditional Medicine, Portland, OR, 1989, p. 21-22

10 Flaws, Bob, "Yin Yang and the Mechanisms of Internal Disease," *Blue Poppy Essays, 1988,* Blue Poppy Press, Boulder, CO, 1988, p. 251-256

11 Jia Kun, op.cit.

12 Song & Yu, op.cit.

13 Han Bai-ling, *Bai Ling Fu Ke (Bai Ling's Gynecology),*

Heilongjiang Peoples Press, Haerbin, 1983, p. 151

The fact that Bensky and Barolet include a formula (She Chuang Zi San) for the treatment of trichimoniasis vaginalis in the *Qu Chong* or parasite-expelling section of *Chinese Herbal Medicine: Formulas and Strategies* underscores and further substantiates the fact that *Chong* can include microbes. Trichimonas is a flagellated protozoan, not a worm.

14   Liang Jian-hui, *A Handbook of Traditional Chinese Dermatology,* trans. by Zhang Ting-liang & Bob Flaws, Blue Poppy Press, Boulder, CO, 1988, p. 17-18

15   Pizzorno & Murray, op.cit., VI:CerDys - 4

16   Flaws, *Sticking to the Point,* op.cit.

17   Tung Ching-chang, *Tung's Acupuncture,* trans. by Decker Palden, revised by Miriam Lee, published by Miriam Lee, Palo Alto, CA, undated

18   Li Su-huai, *Acupuncture Points: 2001,* trans. by M.D. Broffman & Pei Sun F., China Acupuncture Moxibustion Supplies Co, Ltd., Taipei, 1976

19   Liang Rui-jun *et al.,* "Acupuncture Treatment of Cervical Erosion," *Advances in Acupuncture and Anesthesia,* People's Publishing House, Beijing, 1980, p. 96

20   Simonton, O. Carl *et al., Getting Well Again,* J.P. Tharcher, Los Angeles, 1982

21   Lipshultz, op.cit., p. 2

Endnotes to Chapter Four

1. As mentioned above, *Sha Jun* in modern TCM literature simply means anti-microbial. However, in terms of candidiasis, it can be translated as candidacidal since *Jun* means specifically yeast or fungus and *Sha* means to kill. That means we can add the treatment principle to kill yeast or eliminate candida to TCM theory.

2. Trowbridge, John Parks, M.D. & Walker, Marton, D.P.M., *The Yeast Syndrome, How to Help Your Doctor Identify and Treat the Real Cause of Your Yeast-related Illness*, Bantam Books, NY, 1988

3. Katke, Jeffrey, "The Virus Crisis," seminar presented by Metagenics West, Denver, CO, Spring, 1990

4. Zhang Qing-cai & Hsu Hong-yen, *AIDS and Chinese Medicine*, OHAI Press, Long Beach, CA, 1990, p. 171

5. Ibid., p. 173-174

6. Trowbridge & Walker, op.cit., p. 65

7. "Probioplex - Globulin Concentrate from Whey," *Meta Update*, Metagenics West, Denver, Vol. 90, No. 2, p. 1

8. Ibid., p. 1

9. Gyr, K. *et al.*, "The Effect of Oral Pancreatic Enzymes on the Intestinal Flora of Protein Deficient Vervet Monkeys Challenged with Vibrio Cholerae," *American Journal of Clinical Nutrition*, #32, 1979, p. 1592

10. Galland, Leo, M.D. *et al.*, "Giardia Lamblia Infection as a Cause of Chronic Fatigue," *Journal of Nutritional Medicine*, No. 1, 1990, p. 27-31

11	Sung Baek, course materials on Oriental herbalism, Chicago, 1982
12	Braverman, Eric R. & Pfeiffer, Carl C., *The Healing Nutrients Within*, Keats Publishing Inc., New Canaan, CT, 1987, p. 296
13	Ibid., p. 297
14	Stuart, G.A., *Chinese Materia Medica, Vegetable Kingdom*, Southern Materials Center, Inc. Taipei, 1979, p. 181
15	Hsu, Hong-yen *et al.*, *Oriental Materia Medica, A Concise Guide*, OHAI, Los Angeles, 1988, p. 725-726
16	Based on testimonial letters provided by Bioradiance distributor, K'an Herbs Co., and oral communication with Rachel Fresco, practitioner liaison, K'an Herbs Co.
17	Liang Jian-hui, op.cit., p. 45

Endnotes to Chapter Five

1	Zhang & Hsu, op.cit., p. 174
2	For some time I have felt that TCM has short-changed the role of the Large Intestine in health and disease. Western naturopathy and modern environmental medicine both accord the Large Intestine pre-eminence in the cause and treatment of disease. I believe that through an understandiang of classical Inernal Duct theory *vis a vis* the creation of *Wei Qi* and Kidney Yang and the addition of modern insights on candidiasis, amoebiasis, and parasitosis, a much fuller and clinically superior understanding of the pathophysiology and treatment of the Large Intestine can be developed.

3   Tierra, Michael, *Planetary Herbology*, Lotus Press, Sante Fe, NM, 1988, p. 200

4   De Chan, *Shaolin Si Mi Fang Ji Jin (Highlights of Shaolin Monastery's Secret Prescriptions)* ed. by De Qian, Henan Science & Technology Press, Henan, 1983, trans. by Zhang Ting-liang, excerpted in "(Hints From The) Great Monk De Chan For Composing Prescriptions Based on His (60 Years) Personal Experience," *Blue Poppy Essays, 1988*, Blue Poppy Press, op.cit., p. 202

5   Wang Le-ting, excerpted from *Jin Zhen Wang Le Ting (Golden Needle Wang Li-ting)*, trans. by Micheal Helme, appearing in *Timing and the Times*, Blue Poppy Press, Boulder, CO, 1986, p. 140

6   Liang Jian-hui, op.cit., p. 69

7   Pei Zheng-xue, chief editor, *Xue Zheng Lung Ping Shi (Commentary on the Treatise on Blood Disorders)*, People's Hygiene Press, Beijing, 1980, p. 1

8   Ibid., p. 2

9   Riley, David, M.D., "Theory of Homotoxicology," *Biological Therapy, Journal of Natural Medicine*, June, 1990, Vol. VII, No. 3, p. 54

10 Ibid., p. 57

11 Zhang & Hsu, op.cit., p. 17

12 Kaptchuk, Ted, *Jade Pharmacy Product Guide*, Ming Men Design, Aptos, CA, 1988, p. 5-6

13 Seem, Mark, *Acupuncture Imaging*, Thorsons Publishers, Rochester, VT, 1990

14 Matsumoto, Kiiko & Birch, Stephen, *Five Elements and Ten*

Stems, Paradigm Publications, Brookline, MA, undated

15   Xi Yang-jiang, lecture notes, San Francisco, 1983 published in Flaws, *Sticking to the Point*, op.cit., p. 82

16   *The Merck Manual,* op.cit., p. 1825

Endnotes to Chapter Six

1   Liang, Jiang-hui, op.cit., p. 65-68

2   Hsu, Hong-yen & Hsu Chau-shin, *Commonly Used Chinese Herb Formulas With Illustrations,* OHAI, Los Angeles, 1980, p. 489

3   Bensky, Dan & Barolet, Randall, *Chinese Herbal Medicine: Formulas and Strategies,* Eastland Press, Seattle, 1990, p. 206

4   Zhang & Hsu, op.cit., p. 80

5   Hsu & Hsu, op.cit., p. 66

6   Ibid., p. 615

7   Otsuka, Keisetsu *et al., Natural Healing With Chinese Herbs,* compiled & ed. by Hong-yen Hsu, OHAI, Los Angeles, 1982, p. 509

8   Ibid., p. 629

9   Ibid., p. 611

10   Ibid., p. 633

11   Hsu, Hong-yen & Van Benschoten, M.M., *Index of Differentiations for Commonly Used Herb Formulations,* OHAI, Los Angeles, 1984, p. 108

12   Lu, Henry C., *Chinese System of Food Cures*, Sterling Publishing Co., New York, 1986, p. 113

13   Leung, Albert Y. *Chinese Health Remedies*, Universe Books, New York, 1984, p. 144

14   Bensky, Dan & Gamble, Andrew, *Chinese Herbal Medicine: Materia Medica*, Eastland Press, Seattle, 1986, p. 505

Endnotes to Chapter Seven

1   ViraPap tests for men only test the presence of HPV by urethral swab and do not diagnose the prostate for which there is not test comparable to a female Pap for the cervix.

2   *The Merck Manual*, op.cit., p. 250

3   Haywood, Anne M., M.D., "Patterns of Persistent Viral Infections," *New England Journal of Medicine*, Oct. 9, 1986, p. 942

4   Ibid., p. 946

5   Wang Yao-ting, "A Preliminary Discussion of the *Bao Gong, Bao Mai, and Bao Luo*," trans. by Zhang Ting-liang & Bob Flaws, *Blue Poppy Essays 1988*, op.cit., p. 15

6   Chen Zhi-duo, quoted by Wang Yao-ting, op.cit., p. 16

7   Kathleen Belko, D.C., Dipl.Ac., letter to the author, 1990

8   Zhang Jing-yue, quoted by Wang, op.cit., p. 16

9   Tang Zong-hai, quoted by Wang, op.cit., p. 16

10 Elman, op.cit., p. 5

11 Crawford, E. David, "Prostate Cancer: The Ignored Male Disease, Part 2," *Colorado Cancer News*, Vol. VI, No. 5, Dec.

1989, p. 3

12   Ibid., p. 3

13   Ibid., p. 3

14   Nelson *et al.*, op.cit., p. 313

15   Barry, Linda, "Of Jungle Juice and Getting Loose: The Timeless Ritual of Teenage Sex," *The Utne Reader*, No. 40, July/August 1990, p. 94

16   Crawford, op.cit., p 3

17   Crawford, "Prostate Cancer, Part 3," *Colorado Cancer News*, Vol VII, No. 1, February 1990, p. 4

18   Ibid., p. 4

Endnotes to Chapter Eight

1   *Acupuncture Case Histories From China*, ed. by Chen Ji-rui & Nissi Wang, Eastland Press, Seattle, 1988, p. 87-89

Endnotes to Chapter Nine

1   For a concise description of Dr. Yoo Tae-woo's Three Pasttern or Constitution system of diagnosis, see: Eckman, Peter, "Korean Acupuncture," *Traditional Acupuncture Society Journal*, UK, No. 7, April 1990, p. 4-6

2   Flaws, Bob, "You Tae-woo's Three Constitutions and the *Xie Xin* Group of Formulas", forthcoming, *Sheng Chang Herb*

Letter, CA, Winter 1990-91

Endnotes to Chapter Ten

1 Hsu, Hong-yen, "Chinese Herb Therapy for Benign Prostatic Hypertrophy," *OHAI Bulletin*, Los Angeles, Vol. 7, No. 1, June 1982, p. 31-34

2 Ou-Yang Yi, *A Handbook of Differential Diagnosis (&) Treatment*, Vol. 1, trans. by C.S. Cheung, M.D., Harmonious Sunshine Cultural Center, San Francisco, 1987, p. 75

3 Liu, op.cit., p. 307

4 Ou-yang, op.cit., p. 80

5 Ibid., p. 80

6 Ibid., p. 80-81

7 Ibid., p. 75

8 Ibid., p. 81-82

9 Yeung Him-che, *Handbook of Chinese Herbs and Formulas*, Vol. II, self-published, Los Angeles, 1985, p. 46

10 Ou-yang, op.cit., p. 85

11 Ibid., p. 79080

12 Bensky & Barolet, op.cit., p. 201

13 Tung Ching-chang, op.cit.

INDEX

5- flourouacil 22
5-FU 22
5 *Lin* Powder 241
8 Righteous Powder 242
12 *Jing Bie* 163
12 *Jing Jin* 163
12 Regular Channels 163
16 *Luo Mai* 163

A Handbook of Differential Diagnosis (&) Treatment Vol. 1 236
A Handbook of Traditional Chinese Dermatology 80, 124, 171
A Handbook of Traditional Chinese Gynecology 58, 72
A Textbook of Natural Medicine, Vol. I 83
abdominal compresses 72, 79
abdominal cramping 6, 208
abdominal distention after eating 109
abdominal masses 67, 81
abnormal vaginal bleeding
abortions 32
Abutilon 222
Acacia Catechu 74, 75, 79, 133
acanthosis 14, 17, 23, 172
acetic acid 19
aceto-white reaction 19
Acetominophen 23
Acidophilus 76, 106, 135
acne 147, 158
Acquired Kidney Yin and Yang 102
acupuncture viii, 49, 80-82, 86-87, 89-91, 108, 126-127, 158, 162-166, 169, 201, 211-212, 227, 229-230, 233, 253-254
Acupuncture Case Histories from China 201
acute bacterial prostatitis 196
acute gingivostomatitis 116
acute respiratory diseases 116
acute urinary retention 197, 236
adenocarcinoma 197, 198
adenomatous hyperplasia 197
Adenoviruses 188
adrenals 276
adjacent pelvic organs 2
adriamycin 6

adult adenocarcinoma 198
aerobic exercise 212
AG-4 8
aging 39, 106, 197, 203
Ai Gen Er 89
AIDS viii, 37, 53, 60, 63, 69, 111, 133, 143, 212
Alanine 224, 225
Alkeran 6
alcohol 40, 52, 106, 126, 131, 194, 197, 203, 212
Allicin 120, 122
Aloe Vera Juice 114, 135-137
Aloe Vera Plus Herbs 132
Alumen 70, 73, 79
Aluminum Sulphate 270
Alzheimer's disease 189
Ama 155
amenorrhea 67, 87
American Colombo 120
American Ginseng 145
amino acids 82, 83, 137, 225
amoebiasis 40, 99, 109, , 110, 114, 122
amylase 107
Amyotrophic Lateral Sclerosis 189
androscopically visible lesions 21
animal papilloma viruses 10
anogenital warts 173, 176, 179-182, 184, 215
An Tai 145
Anhydrous $MgSO_4$ 269
anti-amoebiasis regime 110
anti-androgens 200
anti-bacterial 104, 152
anti-fungal 104, 114
anti-inflammatory 275
anti-papilloma 75
anti-verrucal 176, 177
anti-viral 67, 72, 73, 76, 113, 126, , 139, 147, 152, 154, 174, 214, 220
antibiotics 99, 100, 104, 106, 199
antibodies 8, 17, 94, 107, 115, 169
anus 19, 21, 25, 76, 127, 172, 189
anxiety 101, 148, 238
Apex Energetics 157, 159, 162, 227
Apex Radicis Angelicae Sinensis 124
appendix of the testes 191

Aquilaria 110, 111, 249
Aquilaria 22 110
Areca 112
Arnica, Inc. 228, 277
Asafoetida 122
Ascendant Liver Yang 118, 226
ascension of the Clear 45, 107, 229
asthma 175
Astra Isatis 85, 117, 118, 214
Astragalus 118, 119, 180, 240
atonic constipation 121
Atractylodes 60, 111, 143, 174
atypical cells 3, 4
Aurantium 113
Avagadro's Number 159
Ayurvedic 111, 112, 137, 144, , 155, 166
Azeopangen 106-108
AZT 164

B Vitamins 156
B_1 228
B_{12} 83, 84, 228
B_6 83
Ba Wei Di Huang Wan 248, 253
Ba Zheng San 241, 242
Bach Flower remedies 158
Bacteria Lactobacilli Acidophili 106
Bacteria Lactobacilli Bifidi 106
Bai Dai 29, 77, 79
Bai Ling Fu Ke 77
Bao Gong 38, 191, 192
Bao Mai 39, 265
Bao Men 192
Barley Fiber 135
Barret *et al.* 15
basement membrane 2, 3
Belamcanda 251
Belko, Kathleen, DC 191
Becker, Thomas M., MD 20
beeswax 74, 182, 183
Bei Xue 87
Bell's palsy 116
Ben Cao 49, 137, 147
Ben Root 58
Beng Lou 97
benign lesion 11
benign prostatic hypertrophy vii, 189, 195, 197, 199-202, 209, 234, 275
Bensky and Barolet 174, 251
Bensky and Gamble 182

Benzoin 183
Beta-carotene 13, 83, 84, 156
Betelnut 112
Bevan, I.S. *et al.* 11
Bian Bing 28, 51, 57, 58, 71, 90, 207
Bian Hou 172
Bian Zheng 27-28, 30, 46, 49, 51, 57-59, 71, 90, 97, 100, 140, 142, 151, 162, 172-173, 185, 201, 207, 214-215, 233, 234, 253
Biao Branch 58
Bichloracetic Acid 22
Bie Xie 222, 242, 243, 248, 251
Bie Xie Fen Qing Yin 248, 251
Bie Xie Shen Shi Tang 242-243
Bifidobacterium Longum 135
bilaminar embryo 190
bilateral orchiectomy 200
bilateral pelvic lymphadenectomy 6
bile 107, 112
bimanual exam 167
Bing Ji 27, 32, 58, 143, 172
Bing Yin 31, 33, 46, 49, 58, 82, 101, 172
Bioenergy Nutrients 85, 236
biopsy 2, 5, 25
Bioradiance 96, 119, 120, 123, 214
biorhythmic cyclicity 17
birth defects 189
Bitter Orange Oil 269
bitter taste 47
bladder 6, 36, 65, 105, 133, 145, 188-191, 197-199, 202, 208, 216-218, 220, 225, 234, 238, 241, 262
bladder cancer 188
bladder outlet obstruction 197, 198
bleeding 29-30, 38, 40, 65-66, 71, 75, 79, 97, 112-113, 133, 153, 238
Blenoxane 6
bleomycin 6
Blessed Thistle 133, 134
Blood Dryness 172
Blood *Lin* 201
Blood Phase 37, 68, 183
bloody discharge 47
Blue Poppy Essays 1988 70
Body Fluids 31, 38, 144, 235
Borax 72, 73, 77, 79
Borax & Alum Powder 73
Borax suppositories 77
borborygmous 177, 225

Boric Acid 77
Borneolum 72, 73, 80
bovine leukemia 119
Bowen's disease 10
Branch symptoms 70, 140
Braverman, Eric R. 115
Broussonetia 118
Brucea 74, 76, 182, 183
Brucea oil 182
Bu An 145
Bu Nei Bu Wai Yin 31-33, 77
Bu Qi 144, 148
Bu Yang 220, 221
Bu Zhong Yi Qi Tang 240
bubonic plague 35
Buddhist monk disease 204
bulbourethral glands 190
Bulbus Alli Sativi 122
Bupleurum 59-63, 68-70, 118, 125, 141-144, 150, 227
Bupleurum & Cinnamon Decoction 68
Bupleurum & Peony Formula 141
Bupleurum & Tang Kuei Formula 141
Bupleurum 12 142
Bupleurum S 150
burning with urination 197
Butternut Bark 134

calcium 135
Calcium Carbonate 135
Calcium Citrate 135
Calm the Stomach Powder 150
cancer 28, 46, 62, 116, 187, 192, 195, 197
cancer-combatting 49
cancer preventive 153, 155
Cancer Root Two 89
Candida Albicans 15, 106
candidiasis 10, 40, 51, 94, 99-101, 108, 109, 119, 132, 137, 212, 271
candicidal regime 103, 106
candidicide 105
carbuncle/dermatosis 175
carcinogens 11
carcinoma in situ 1-5, 8, 262
Cardomom 114
Carson *et al.* 17
catheterization 199, 200
cauliflower-shaped lesions 19
Caulis Akebiae Mutong 124-126, 178,

181, 235, 237, 239, 242-243, 250
cauterization 5, 23, 182
cavernous lesions 46
cell-mediated immunity 18
cellular atypia 17
cellular genes 11
cellular immunity 16
central nervous system 116, 190
cervical canal 191
cervical cancer 1-3, 6-10, 12, 13, 16, 27-31, 46, 47, 62, 63, 114, 167, 168, 210, 213
cervical dysplasia vii, viii, ix, 1-10, 12, 13, 16, 26-28, 30, 32-35, 37, 39, 46, 48, 51, 53, 57, 64, 71-73, 79, 83, 86, 87, 90, 94, 97, 100, 114, 117, 136, 140, 150, 166, 167, 168, 171, 187, 201, 202, 210, 213, 219, 232
cervical erosion 90
cervical intraepithelial neoplasia x, 1, 3, 24, 26
cervical papilloma 38
cervical pathology 11
cervical powders 72
cervical scarring 6
cervicitis 116
cervix 1-6, 11, 19, 20, 22, 25, 38, 43, 72, 76, 78, 89, 93, 108, 156, 158, 187-189, 191-192, 261, 270
CFIDS 109
Chai Hu Gui Zhi Tang 68, 70, 140, 142, 143
Chamber of Essence 192
Channel & Collateral Patterns 163
Channel Divergences 163
Channel Sinews 163
Chaparral 73, 135, 136, 182, 220-222
Chaste Tree Berries 149
Chelidonum Majus 159
chemotherapy 6
Chen Xiang San 248-249
chest distention 47
Chest Qi 34, 148
Cheung, C.S., Dr. 60
Chi Bai Dai 29
Chi Ke 113
chicken pox 164, 194
Chih-ko 113
Chih-shih 113
Children of Your Own: The Mojzis

297

Method 55, 56
Chinese disease category 27, 30, 108, 210, 207
Chinese menopathy 58
Chionathus Virginicus 159
chlamydia 10, 15, 37, 195
Chlamydia Trachomatis 10, 15
Chlorotene 83
cholera 35
cholesterol 153, 154, 275-276
Chong 32-33, 38, 60, 77, 100, 105, 108-110, 112-113, 122-123, 137, 164-166, 264
Chong and *Ren* 32, 60, 166
Chong Mai/Bao Mai 38
chronic bacterial prostatitis 196, 199
chronic Damp Heat skin leasions 180
Chronic Fatigue Immune Deficiency Syndrome 109
Chronic Fatigue Syndrome, The Hidden Epidemic 276
chronic non-bacterial prostatitis 196, 199
chronic respiratory complaints 175
chronic skin conditions 180
chronic viral infections viii, x, 110, 227
Chou Xin Yin 242-243
Chun Ze Tang 240
Ci Hou 171
Cicada 180
CIN 1, 3-4, 6-8, 11-12, 14, 22-27, 31-33, 36-39, 51-54, 56-59, 64, 72-74, 78, 81, 87-91, 101, 103, 114-115, 123, 129-130, 139, 156, 167-168, 187, 213, 227-230, 269-270
CIN 1-3 269-270
Cinnabaris 72
Cinnamon and Hoelen Formula 244
Cinnamon and Poria Pills 244
CIS 1, 3-5, 74, 270
Class I-V 3, 4
Clear the Heart Lotus Seed Drink 239
Clear the Lungs, Purge Fire Pills 235
Clear Yang 103, 105
Cleves, Margaret 6
clitoris 25
cloaca 189-191
Cloves 133
CMV viii, 102, 157, 188, 210, 227, 276
Cnidium Monnierum 104

cockcrow diarrhea 247
co-enzymes 82
co-factors 12, 82
CO_2 laser 5
coccyx 54
Cod Liver Oil 74, 75, , 156
Codonopsis 62, 69, 104, 110, 111, 117, 118, 126, 145, 223
coffee enemas 81, 105
Coix 173-177, 180-181, 243
Coix Combination 174, 175
Coix Decoction 174
Cold Injury 35
Colloidum Frasera 121
Colon Care formula 132, 134, 135
colon cleansing 131, 132, 137, 138
colposcopy 2, 21, 22, 24, 25
colposcopically visible lesions 95
Comfrey Root 75, 78, 79, 183
Comfrey Root Douche 78
Commanding points 87
commensal fungus 99
Commentary on the Treatise on Blood Disorders 154
common warts 171, 172, 181, 182
Compound Dang Gui Injectible 228
Concha Ostreae 126, 179
condoms 94, 95, 167, 195, 232
Conduct Red Powder 239
condyloma 18, 23, 94, 193, 269-270
condylomata acuminatum 23
condylomata 15, 18, 19, 22-24, 169
condylomatous growth pattern 2
cone biopsy 5
Congealed Blood 122
Congested Fluids in the Middle 146
conization 5
conjunctivitis 116
connective tissue 190
constitutional imbalances 139, 163
Coptis 121, 125, 215
Coptis Purge Fire Tablets 125, 215
corns 175
Cornu Bubali 68
Cornu Rhinoceri 68
Cortex Ailanthi Altissimae 64, 65
Cortex Cinnamomi 248, 250
Cortex Juglandis Cinerae 133
Cortex Magnoliae Officinalis 150, 237
Cortex Meliae Azerdach 110, 112

Cortex Phellodendri 104, 119, 125, 180, 243-244, 247-248
Cortex Radicis Lycii 239
Cortex Radicis Moutan 60, 126, 178, 223, 244-245, 247, 248
Cortex Tabebuiae Impetiginosae 105
cortisone 276
Cou Li 80
Crawford, Dr. E. David 192-194, 199
creation and transformation 102
Crohn's disease 189
cryosurgery 4-6, 22
CV 1 126, 228
CV 2 228
CV 5-7 218
CV 8 80
cyclophamide 6
Cyperus 141, 147-149
cystitis 100, 116, 202, 254
cytomegalovirus viii
Cytoxan 6

Da Heng 217
Da Huang Mu Dan Pi Tang 245
Dai Xia 29, 30, 38, 48, 58, 61, 64-66, 75, 77-79, 86, 87, 97, 100, 133, 134, 153
Dai Xia Douche 79
Damiana 221
Damp Cold Obstruction & Stagnation of Blood 241-244 Damp foods 51, 52, 203
Damp Heat 29-30, 37-40, 42, 48-49, 61, 64-67, 71, 73, 76-79, 84, 100, 103, 105, 107, 109, 117-119, 122, 124-125, 134, 136, 145, 153, 172-173, 177, 179-180, 183, 202-208, 212-214, 216-225, 229, 235, 239, 241-243
Damp Heat Accumulating in the Bladder 202-203, 241
Damp Heat *Lin* 219, 225
Damp Hot Toxins 49, 79
Damp Toxins 49, 105
Dampness 29-30, 32-33, 37-40, 42, 48, 52-54, 59-61, 63- 64, 69, 71-77, 85-86, 98, 100, 103-111, 114, 118-121, 123-126, 130, 133-134, 138, 140, 143-150, 153-155, 166, 173-176, 178, 180, 195, 237-239, 241-245, 248-249, 251-252
Dan Tian 55, 102, 192
Dan Zhi Xiao Yao San 60-62, 85, 141, 142
Dandelion 63
Dang Gui 146
Dao 29, 37, 139, 234, 238-239
Dao Chi San 238-239
dark field, live cell microscopy 101
deep relaxation xii, 56, 57, 86, 138, 162, 212, 213, 230
Defensive Qi 44
Deficiency cold symptoms 247
Deficiency Heat 42, 209, 212, 241, 245-247
Deficiency Heat in the Lower Burner 241, 245
Deficient Yin Fire 118
depletion of Yin Humor 37
depression 6, 47, 84, 100, 101, 103, 120, 134, 136, 144, 149, 221
Depressive Liver Fire 41, 149, 203, 213
Depressive Liver Heat 30, 41, 61, 86
Dermomyositis 189
DES 21
descension of the Turbid 45, 107, 138, 151, 185, 229
detection by DNA probe 19
Dharmananda, Subhuti 68
diabetes 189
Dian 30
diarrhea 6, 66, 82, 100, 107, 109, 112-113, 133, 173, 226, 238, 247
diet viii, xii, 40, 48, 51-53, 57, 91, 99, 106, 130-132, 138, 162, 181, 194, 203, 212, 276, 271
dietary therapy 51, 53, 86
digestion 40, 54, 56, 101, 106, 108, 130, 148, 151, 166, 177, 213
digestive disturbance 109
digestive enzymes 107, 108
digital rectal exam 196, 198, 199, 204
Dioscorea 118
disease mechanisms 27-30, 35, 143, 150, 202, 234, 239, 241, 268
Dispelling Swelling Pills 223
disruption in the flow and patency of Qi 31
disseminated disease of the newborn 116
distal urethra 190
dizziness 246
DNA 8-11, 14, 18-21, 24, 25, 95, 96,

299

168, 214, 227
DNA hybridization 20
DNA probes 18, 20
DNA typing 9
douches 72, 78
Dragon Gall Liver Purging Decoction 124
dragon spirits 91
Drak Sum Gonpo 91
dribbling urination 202, 209
Dried Aloe Vera Juice 114
Dry Phlegm Cough 75
dry skin 175
dry stools 46
Du 48-49, 65, 77, 122-123, 137, 153, 178, 194, 264, 268
Dual Kidney Yin & Yang Deficiency 247
Dual Liver/Kidney Deficiency 226
duct of the epididymus 190
ductus deferens 191
duration of remedial treatment 96
Dynamic Warrior 253
dysbiosis 109, 110, 112, 114
dysentery-like disorders 64
dysmenorrhea 30, 55-56, 65, 86-88, 100, 144, 147, 149, 158, 244
dyspareunia 55
dysuria 6, 153, 196, 250

E-400 Selenium 253
E. Coli 107
Eagle Marketing 132, 135, 137, 277
early first intercourse 7
early periods 30, 158
EBV viii, 11, 102, 157, 188, 210, 227, 276
EBV shedding 11
ecchymotic patches 208
ectoderm 189, 190
eczema herpeticum 116
edema 66, 222, 225, 236
ejaculate 20, 231
ejaculation 224, 226, 231
ejaculatory duct 191
elastases 107
electrocoagulation 4
elevated serum cholesterol 276
elimination 54, 56, 107, 155
ELISA 107

embryonic mesoderm 190
emotional irritability 47
emotional stress 48, 143, 194, 204, 208, 238, 250
emotional upset 31, 41, 56
endocervical canal 2, 5
endocervical curettage 2, 5
endoderm 189-191
endometrioma 88
endometriosis 55, 178
enemas 72, 81, 105, 255
enlarged prostate 220, 221
Enterococcus Faecium 135
enuresis 205
environmental factors 7, 192
environmental medicine 109
environmental pollution 99
enzymes 82, 83, 107, 108, 275
Ephedra, Forsythia, & Phaseolus Decoction 236
epidemiology 12, 18, 26
epidermis 14, 190
epidermodysplasia verruciformis 10, 16
epigastric pain 139
Epimedium 118, 226
epithelial spicules 23
epithelium 1, 2, 5, 9, 14, 15, 190, 191
epoophoron 191
Epsom salt baths 105
Epstein-Barr virus viii, 11, 188, 189
Er Chen Tang Jia Wei 237
erythema multiforme 116
escarosis 74, 76, 182-183, 270
escarotic therapy 74, 76, 78, 93-94, 269-270
esophagus 10, 89
Essence 35, 37-39, 44, 55, 75, 84-85, 102, 118-119, 134, 138, 151-152, 179-180, 191-194, 205-206, 212-214, 218-226, 229, 231, 253
Essence Chamber Tablets 214, 219, 220, 222-225, 253
Essential Book of Traditional Chinese Medicine, The 68, 236
eustachian tube
Evil Heat 30-31, 54, 69, 103, 142, 145, 203, 206, 213, 226, 234, 267
Evil Heat in the Lungs 103
Evil Qi 37, 44, 48, 86, 91, 117, 127, 154, 174, 175, 179, 180

Evil Spirit Gates 44
Evodia 121
Excess Bile 112
Excess Heat 35, 42, 85, 253
excessive leukorrhea 47
excessive liquids 52
Excessive Menstruation 64
excessive perspiration 238
excessive sex 39
Excrementum Bombycis Mori 243
Excrementum Trogopterori Seu Pteromi 70
exercise xii, 41, 48, 51, 53-57, 86, 138, 162
Exhaustion of Blood and *Jing* Essence 35
Exhaustion *Lin* 202
exteriorization 23, 164, 165, 180
exteriorized pathogen 23
External causes 31, 32
External Invasions 48
External Medicine 49
External pathogens 33, 37
external therapies 51
Extra points 80, 87
Extractum Dessicatum Herbae Aloes 111, 114
Extractum Herbae Cum Radice Isatidis 125
Extractum Semenis Curcubitaceae 224
extravasation 113

facial edema 236
failure of immune response 24
fallopian tubes 5, 191
False Cold 54
false negative Paps 20
False Unicorn 221
Fang Ji Xue 57, 235
Fang Lao 203
fasting 40
fatigue 39, 101, 109, 202-203, 231, 246-247, 276
FDA 20
Feldenkrais floor work 56
Female Balance 157
female hormones 200
Ferenczy, Dr. Alex, 21
Ferenczy *et al.* 9
Ferric Sulphate 269

Ferula Galbaniflua 122
ferulic esters 275
Fetal Leakage 38
Fetal Palace 192
Fetal Toxins 194
fever 6, 40, 113, 116, 165, 196, 197
fever blisters 116
fibrocystic breasts 64, 65
Fieldmint 60, 61, 136
filiform warts 171
Finch, Jack 193
Five *Lin* 241
Fire Toxins 49, 63, 65, 122, 182
Five Elements and Ten Stems 163
Five Fruits Pills 152
Five *Lin* 201
Five Peels Powder 152
Five Phase dyscrasias 163
Five Phase theory 29
Five Phase *Ke* cycle 52, 81
Five Transport Points 229
Flaring of Deficiency Fire 226
flat warts 171, 172
flatulence 82, 100, 109, 225
Flaxseed Oil 225, 226
Flos Caryophylli 133
Flos Lonicerae 68, 178, 179
Flos Schizonepetae 180, 181
Flos Trifolii 133, 134
fluey feelings 165
fluted tongue 47
Folic Acid 13, 78, 83, 84, 156, 184
Folium Cycasis Revolutae 66
Folium Isatidis 68
Folium Menthae Piperitae 136
Folium Perillae 236-237
Folium Plantaginis 132, 133
Foot *Jue Yin* 115, 118
Four (Methods of) diagnosis 28, 101, 161, 162, 210, 229
Four Counterflows 54
Four Ingredient Decoction 63
Four Medicinal Oil Paste 74
Four Stages 36, 198
Frasera 120, 121
Free & Easy Powder 59, 60
frequent miscarriage 88
frigidity 100
Fringe Tree 159
Front Mu Points 217, 219

Fructificatio Ganodermae Lucidi 152
Fructificatio Lentini 152
Fructificatio Polypori Mylittae 110, 112
Fructificatio Tremellae 152
Fructus Amomi Cardamomi 104, 111, 114
Fructus Arctii 181
Fructus Aridus Euphorbiae Longanae 62, 65
Fructus Broussonetiae 66, 117, 118
Fructus Bruceae Javanicae 64, 74, 182, 183
Fructus Citri Seu Ponciri 110, 113, 143, 237, 250
Fructus Cnidii Monnieri 79, 104
Fructus Corni 247-248
Fructus Forsythiae 125
Fructus Gardeniae 60, 124-126, 180, 235, 242-243
Fructus Germinatus Hordei 150
Fructus Immaturus Citri Seu Ponciri 70-71, 113, 243
Fructus Ligustri Lucidi 223
Fructus Lycii 117
Fructus Myristicae Fragrantis 111, 113
Fructus Pruni Mume 110, 111
Fructus Quisqualis Indicae 110, 112
Fructus Serenoae Serrulatae 220, 224, 225
Fructus Terminaliae Chebulae 110, 112
Fructus Viticis Agnus-casti 144, 149
Fructus Zizyphi Jujubae 62, 69, 144, 147, 171, 240
Fruit Pectin 135
Fu Fang Dang Gui Zhu She Ye 228
Fu Fang Zi Cao Gao 183
Fu Ke 58, 77, 88, 171
Fu Ke Xue 88
Fu Ling 42, 244
Fu Liu 165
Fu Mai 42, 210
Fu Xie 36-39, 42, 43, 48, 161, 187, 210
Fu Zheng 74, 76, 78, 106, 155
Fu Zheng suppositories 78
fumigation 127
Fumitory 122
Fundamentals of Chinese Medicine 67
fungal diseases 176
fungal infection 20
fungi 113, 122, 228, 272

Gallbladder 66, 84, 120-122, 124, 133, 136, 144, 149, 216-218, 226, 235, 264, 266-267
Gambir 118, 119, 214
Gan Qi 41
ganglionitis 115
Ganoderma 152, 153
Gao Yao Feng 80
Gardenia & Hoelen Formula 241
Garlic 122, 137
Garuda 91
Gastrodia 141
Gate of the *Bao* 192
Gate position 103
Gates of Qi 44
Ge-132 85, 226
gemmotherapeutics 158
genetic predisposition 16
genital fluxes 118
genital tract 10, 14, 16, 24, 94
genital tract candidiasis 94
genital wart virus 73
genital warts 14-16, 18, 25, 95, 96, 171-172, 182, 213, 215, 233
genitalia viii, 8, 20, 34, 37, 66, 85, 96, 99, 114, 116, 117, 118, 123-125, 127, 210, 214, 233
genome 11, 14, 17
Getting Well Again 92
Ginger 60, 61, 69, 81, 111
Ginger tea 81
Ginseng 62, 69, 143, 145, 177, 227, 239-240
glands of the prostate 190
Glutamic Acid 225
Glycine 224, 225, 269
glycogen 276
Goldenseal 121
Golden Rod 225
gonorrhea 15, 178, 195
Gotu Kola 143, 144
Gotu Kola 15 Formula 143
granulomatous prostatitis 198
greasy tongue coating 108, 237, 241
Greater Celandine 159, 182
greater vestibular glands
Green Citrus Peel 63
Grifola 153
groin 66, 118, 179
gross condylomata 15, 19

Ground Mallow 222
Gu 44, 126, 228
Guan 103, 164, 165, 236
Guan Chong 164, 165
Guar Gum 135
Gui Lai 80
Gui Men 44
Gui Pi Tang 61, 62
Gui Pi Tang Jia Chai Hu 62
Gummum Acaciae 132
Gummum Benzoin 183
Gummum Galbani 120, 122
Gummum Olibani 80
gynecological neoplasms 61
Gynecological Points 88
Gypsum 181, 236

H_2O_2 137
Haemophilus Ducreyi 15
Haemophilus Saunus 107
Hahnemann, Samuel 156
Hai Bao 253-254
Han Bai-ling 77
Han Liang Pai 35
Hansen *et al.* 9
Harmonizing formula 150
Hatch, Kenneth D. 24
Hatha yoga 56
Haywood, Anne M. 188, 189
He Fang 150
headache 144, 146
Health World 275
Heart 34, 38, 47-48, 60-62, 65, 67-70, 84, 103, 111, 113, 121-122, 144-149, 152-154, 176-177, 180, 206-209, 216-218, 221, 234, 238-239, 242, 254, 265, 268
heart attacks 154, 206
Heart Blood 34, 47, 48, 61, 62, 148, 152
Heart Blood/Spleen Qi Deficiency 47, 61
Heart Blood Deficiency 48
Heart Fire 238
Heart *Shen* 68
Heart/ Small Intestine Fire 209
Heart Spirit 60, 113, 148, 154
heat in the chest and upper back 238
Heat in the Five Centers 209
Heavenly Water 143
hematuria 153, 196-198, 201, 208, 236
Heng Gu 228

hepatitis 116, 188, 189, 276
Herba Achilleae Millefolii 269
Herba Agrimoniae 70, 71
Herba Artemesiae Capillaris 104
Herba Baijiangcao 176
Herba Cardui Benedicti 133
Herba Cum Radice Asari 236
Herba Cum Radice Impatientis Pallidae 120, 121
Herba Cum Radice Taraxaci Mongolici 63
Herba Dendrobii 243
Herba Dianthi 242, 250
Herba Ephedrae 174, 175, 236
Herba Epimedii 117
Herba Fumariae Officinalis 120, 122
Herba Houttuyniae Cordatae 104
Herba Lophatheri Gracilis 125, 239
Herba Menthae 59, 60, 136, 237
Herba Passiflorae Incarnatae 143, 144
Herba Patriniae 175, 176, 223
Herba Polygoni Avicularis 242
Herba Pyrrosiae 249
Herba Selaginellae Doerderleinii 64, 66
Herba Solani Lyrati 63, 65
Herba Solidaginis 224, 225
Hering, Constantine 228
herpes genitalia viii, 8, 37, 85, 99, 114, 117, 123-125, 210, 214, 233
herpes labialis 116
herpes outbreaks 53-54, 57, 63-64, 69-70, 118, 122-123, 126, 134, 142, 154, 214, 219
herpes progenitalis 116
herpes simplex II viii, 10, 33, 114, 116
herpetic whitlow 116
Herxheimer reaction 105
hesitancy and intermittency of stream 197
Hidden Blood Rash 180
Hidden Evil 36, 37, 42, 43, 45, 48, 74, 95, 98, 115, 151, 180, 187
Hidden Evils 36-38, 43, 154, 161, 193, 229
Hidden Paper-like Herb 42
hidden pulse 42, 210
Hippocrates 92
HIV viii, 16, 17, 37, 43, 53, 93, 102, 107, 119, 120, 123, 136, 152, 164, 165, 188, 210, 276

Hlavaty, Vaclav 55
Hoelen 153, 240-241, 244
homeopathic medicines 157, 158, 160, 161
homeopathically adjusted allopathic medications 158
homeopathically adjusted orthomoleculars 158
homeopathy 156-162, 227, 228
homotoxicological remedies 129, 158, 227
homotoxicology 156, 158-160, 212, 227
Honey-baked Licorice 60, 148
hormonal fluctuations 100, 197
hormone inhibitors 200
horny cornification 178
Horse Gold Water 254
Horse Quick Water 254
Hot *Lin* 201
Hot Stagnant Blood 41
Hot Toxins 35, 48, 49, 79, 214
Hot Urinary Disturbance 153
Houttuynia 104
HPV 8-12, 14-27, 33, 37-39, 43, 45, 48, 74, 93, 94-96, 98, 115-119, 123, 129, 139, 157, 158, 165, 167-169, 171, 183-185, 187-193, 195, 205, 210-211, 214, 228, 232-233, 243
HPV 16 or 18 21
HPV 18 21
HPV 6, 11, and 42 21
HPV antigens 16
Hsu, Hong-yen 47, 62, 122, 234
Hsu and Hsu 175, 177-179
Hsu and Van Benschoten 180
HSV-2 antigen 8
Hu Chang San 244-245
Hua 41-44, 102, 108, 119, 155, 208, 241, 249, 252
Hua Re 41
Hua Shi Tang 252
Huan Chao 88
Huang Dai 29, 78, 79
Huang Jin Qing Fei Yin 235
Huang Shu 218
Hui Yin 126, 127, 228
human immuno-deficiency virus viii
human papilloma virus 8, 9, 18, 33, 115
human wart virus 9
Hun 84, 145

Hydrastis 120, 121, 269
Hydrastis Tincture 269
Hydrangea 220-222
Hydrogen Peroxide 137, 138
hydrotherapy 254-255
hydroxyuria 6
Hyperactive *Ming Men Huo* 119
hyperplasia 14, 19, 197
hypertension 118, 119, 206
hypnotherapy 92
hypotonic buttock and abdominal muscles 54
hysterectomy 5, 6

iatrogenesis 25
immune response 12, 18, 23, 24, 59, 98, 169, 171, 184, 197
immune system 12, 15-18, 43, 45, 59, 94, 98-100, 102, 127, 129, 162, 184, 185, 195, 227, 232, 276
immune system incompetence 15
immunocompromise 21
Immunosode 157, 227
Immunotox 157
Imperial Grace Formulary of the Tai Ping Era 140
impotence 172, 200
incantation 90, 91
incomplete emptying 197
incontinence 200, 247
increased sexual activity 193, 194
indigestion 109, 110
Indigo 66, 72-74, 76
inguinal hernia 254
infantile eczema 194
infectious soft warts 171
infertility 54, 87, 88, 100
inflammation of the cervix 93
inflammation of the prostate 195
injury to the *Chong* and *Ren* 32
Inner Evils 164
inner tympanic membrane 190
Inside to Outside 36, 164, 174, 194
insomnia 40, 47, 144, 146, 154, 206, 238, 246
Insubstantial Stagnation 141
integrated Chinese-Western medicine x
interferon injection 23, 24, 184
intermediate mesoderm 190
Internal Accumulation of Evil Heat 31

Internal causes 31
Internal Dampness 52
Internal Duct of the Triple Heater 102
internal environment of the pelvis 54, 97
internal environmental factors 7
Internal Evil Heat imploded within 69
Internal Gate of the Triple Heater 45, 165
Internal Heat 52, 54, 57, 70
Internal Injury (due to the Seven Passions) 31
Internal Stirring of Wind 119
Intestinal Abscess 175, 176
intestinal bacteria 135
intra-anal digital massage of the prostate 254
intravaginal applicator 22, 72, 76, 78
Intrinsi B₁ /Folate 83
involuntary twitching 230
irregular menstruation 88, 97, 146, 147, 150
irregular vaginal bleeding 30
Isatis Cooling Formula 125, 215
Isatis Tinctorius 72
itching 67, 88, 134
IUDs 31

Jade Gate Pea 127
Jade Pharmacy 161
Javier, R. T., *et al.* 11
Jewelweed 121
Jia Kun 29, 31-33, 38, 70, 155
Jie Du 49, 65, 77, 122, 123, 137, 153, 178
Jie Jie Wan 202, 223, 253
Jin 33, 35, 56, 76, 79, 84, 101, 155, 161, 163, 166, 172, 225, 235, 248, 251-254
Jin Gui Yao Lue 161, 225, 248
Jin Sinews 56, 76, 84, 172
Jin Zi-jou 34
Jin-Yuan Dynasties 35, 155
Jing 30, 35-36, 38-39, 44-45, 48, 58, 64, 75, 79-80, 84-86, 94-95, 97, 102-103, 106, 118-119, 130, 134, 138, 147, 151, 152, 154, 159, 161, 163, 172, 176, 179-180, 191-194, 202, 205-206, 212, 216-219, 220, 224-229, 231, 234, 265-266
Jing Fang 161
Jing Luo 44, 163

Jing Luo Pattern identification 163
Jing She 192, 220
Jing Sou Bu Li 202
Jing Xing Ru Fang Zhang Tong 58, 97
Job's Tears 173
joint pain 196
Jue Yin 41, 115, 118, 145, 149, 222
Jun 33, 77, 90, 100, 109, 113, 123

K'an Herbs 120, 124, 141, 214, 253, 277
Kai Kit Wan 202, 223, 253
Kalenite Herbal formula 132
Kampo 160, 161, 174-176
Kang Ai 49, 63, 64, 122, 134, 154
Kaptchuk, Ted 141, 161
Katke, Jeffrey, Dr. 102
keratoconjunctivitis 116
Ki 10 126
Ki 11 228
Ki 16 218
Ki 7 165
Kidney Deficiency 202, 205, 208-209, 226, 247
Kidney Essence 37, 38
Kidney Excess 215, 218
Kidney *Jing* 38, 39, 85, 95, 103, 118, 205
Kidney Qi 103, 112, 203, 205, 221-222, 246
kidney stones 254
Kidney Yang 37, 45, 84-85, 102-103, 133-134, 165, 176, 205-206, 209, 212, 217-218, 221, 246, 248-249
Kidney Yang Deficiency 102, 205, 221, 246, 248
Kidney Yin 34, 47, 102, 118, 194, 205, 209, 222, 226, 246-248, 265
Kidney Yin Deficiency 47, 205, 222, 246
Kidney/Bladder 36
Kidneys 38, 44-45, 66, 69, 85, 102, 106, 111-113, 133, 138, 154, 173, 203, 206, 212, 216-218, 221-222, 228, 245, 264-265, 268
knee and lumbar soreness and pain 47
koilocytotic changes 14
Korean medicine 113
Krebs cycle catalysts 158
Kryzanwska, Romana 55

305

l-Alanine 224
l-Glutamine 224
l-Glycine 224
labia majora 127
Lacca Sinica Exiccata 67
Lactobacillus Acidophilus 76, 135
Lactobacillus Casei Var. Rhamnosis 135
Laminaria 118
Lancaster and Jenson 10, 16, 17
Lao Lin 202, 207
Large Intestine 36-37, 45, 64, 66-67, 75, 81, 101-103, 104-108, 111-114, 121-122, 130-131, 132-134, 136-137, 145, 165, 176-179, 212, 216-218, 220-221, 225, 251, 264
Large Intestine function 102, 106, 112, 130, 212
Larrea 73
Larson *et al.* 9
laser cauterization 5, 23
laser surgery 5, 7, 22
laser vaporization 25, 182
latent infection stage 9
latent pathogens 36
latent stage 12, 39
lateral mesoderm 190
leakage from the Intestines 112, 113
leakage of Lung Qi 112
Lectures of Surgery in Chinese Medicine 47
left *Chi* 103
Lentinus 152, 153
leukorrhea 38, 46-48, 87, 88, 176
Leung, Albert Y. 181
leuprolide 200
Levelling & Dispersing Elixir 70
Li Dong-yuan 44, 266
Li Qi 32, 33, 111, 113, 138, 144, 172, 205
Li Shi-cai 101
Li Shi-zhen's system 101
Li Su-huai 87
Liang, Jian-hui 171, 172
Liang Rui-jun *et al.* 90
Lichenificatio Usneae 269
Licorice 60, 69, 111, 148, 174-175, 180, 183, 242
Lift Anus Muscle 127
Lignum Aquilariae Agallochae 110, 111, 249
Ling Zhi mushroom 152
Linoleic Acid 225
Linseed Oil 225
lipase 107
lipid-coated viruses 276
Lipshultz, Larry I. 17
Liquid Folate 78, 156
liquid meal replacement 103
Lithospermum & Oyster Shell Decoction 179
Lithospermum Ointment 182, 183
lithotherapeutics 158
Liu Wan-su 31, 35, 41
Liu Wei Di Huang Wan 223, 246-247, 253
Liu Xie 31
Liu Yan-chi 37, 236
Liv 2 126
Liv 8 126
Liver 25, 30-31, 34, 41, 47-48, 52-56, 59-61, 63-70, 74-75, 79-82, 84-87, 93-94, 98, 102-103, 105, 108, 111-112, 114, 118-122, 124-125, 133-134, 136-138, 140-141, 143-147, 149-151, 153-156, 165-166, 172-174, 180, 183, 190, 202-204, 208, 212-213, 215-218, 220-222, 224-226, 235, 239, 241242, 250-251, 276
Liver Blood Deficiency 119, 172, 173, 242
Liver Blood/Kidney Yin Deficiency 47
Liver Channel 34, 64, 65, 84, 125, 145, 172, 183
Liver Congestion/Qi Stagnation 202, 203, 208
Liver Deficiency 172
Liver Heat 30, 41, 48, 53, 61-62, 86, 94, 136, 140, 147
Liver Heat/Heart Blood Insufficiency 62
Liver Meridian 34
Liver Qi 41, 48, 52-54, 56, 59, 61, 69, 82, 87, 93, 98, 103, 118, 136, 140-141, 144-147, 149-150, 165, 203-204, 208, 213, 250
Liver Qi Congestion 41, 140, 146, 203
Liver Qi/Liver Heat 48, 140
Liver Wood 60, 111
Liver/Lung cough 121
Liver/Spleen Disharmony 61

Liver/Spleen dyscrasia 143
Liver/Stomach Channel Cold Phlegm disorders 121
local immune response 23
local points 87, 127
local vitamin injection 184
localized prostate cancer 200
Long Bi 201, 207, 219, 229
Long Dan Xie Gan Tang 124, 214
long term fatigue 39
loose stools 101, 107, 109, 142, 226, 253
Lotus Seed Combination 239
low back pain 56, 196
low cholesterol diet 276
low serum beta-carotene 13
lower abdominal pain 30, 87
Lower Burner 36-39, 41, 48, 55, 61, 67, 69, 76, 79, 86, 103-105, 111-113, 118-119, 124-125, 132-134, 173, 175, 176, 178-179, 195, 203-206, 212, 217, 220-222, 225, 234, 239, 241-245, 247, 249-250, 266
Lower *Jiao* 104, 221
lower socio-economic status 193, 194
Lu 11 164
Lu and Needham 45
Lu, Henry C. 181
lumbago 47
lumbar soreness/sprain 47, 254
lumena of the Channels 251
Lung Deficiency 209
Lung Heat 84, 121, 134, 209, 235-236
Lung Qi 52, 112, 164, 165, 174
Lung Qi's empowerment of Large Intestine function 112
Lung Yin 34, 237-238
Lung Yin Deficiency 237
Lungs 34, 36, 65, 68-70, 75, 102-103, 111-113, 121, 133, 134, 143, 145-148, 153-154, 173-175, 180, 216-218, 221, 225-226, 234-237, 239, 251, 264, 266
Luo 44, 67, 71, 163, 172, 265
Lycium 118
lymph vessel walls 190
lymphadenitis 179
lymphatic system 3, 228
lymphatic tissue 190
Lymphotox 157, 227

Ma Huang Lian Qiao Chi Dou Tang 236
Ma Huang Yi Gan Tang 175
Ma Jin Shui 253-254
Ma Kuai Shui 253-254
Macrobiotic 53, 131, 271
macules 15, 19
Male Balance 227
male sexual partners 167
malignant cells 3
malignant skin diseases 179
malnourishment of the *Jin* 172
Malva 222
mammary glands 190
mammograms 198
Manaka's Ion Pumping Cords 229
Massa Medica Fermentata 108
Masochistic 217
massage 165, 166, 212, 230, 254
mastoid air cells 190
Matsumoto and Birch 163
Mayway Trading Co. 141, 277
measles 153, 164, 194
Medical Revelations 252
Medicine Wheel ix, xi
meditation 91
Medulla Junci Effusi 242
Medulla Tetrapanacis 244, 252
melancholy 47
Melia 112
meningoencephalitis 116
menopathies 54-56, 58, 86, 97, 98, 101, 108
menopause 5, 21, 206
menorrhagia 29, 64, 88
menstrual cycle 48, 59, 98, 151
menstruation 58, 61, 64, 71, 73-74, 76, 80, 86, 88, 93, 97, 146-147, 150, 166-167, 192
Merck Manual, The 25
mesoderm 189, 190
mesonephric duct 190
mesopharangeal cancers 66
Metagenics 77, 83, 103, 106-107, 156, 224, 253, 277
metastases 198
metastatic ovarian and liver tumors 25
metastatic prostate cancer 200
methotrexate 6
metrorrhagia 29
Mi Fang 120

miasms 194
micronutrient deficiencies 12
microscopic visible detection 19
Middle Burner 36, 42, 118, 134, 151, 222, 239, 266
middle ear 190
middle-aged men 118, 202, 212
migraines 100
milking the prostate 254
minerals 82, 83, 85, 120, 137, 157, 224
Ming Men 69, 70, 94, 111, 113, 119, 136, 149, 176, 206, 263-268
Ming Men Fire 94, 111, 113, 149, 206, 118
Ming Men Huo 70, 119
minor vestibular gland excision 24
Mirabilitum 178
mixed Excess/Deficiency Damp Heat 42
moderate dysplasia 2-5, 85, 187, 270
Mojzis, Ludmila 54, 56
Mojzis Method 55, 56
monilia 94
Moon Flow Before Schedule 30
Moutan 60-61, 68, 126, 141, 177-178, 221, 223, 244-245, 247-248
Moutan & Gardenia Free & Easy Powder 60
Mowrey, David B, PhD. 275
moxa 127
MS 93, 189
Mu Fu 87
Mu Xiang Shun Qi Wan 150
Multigenics 83
multi-partner sexual activity 194
multiple sexual partners 7, 21, 33, 194, 196, 210
Mume 110-113
muscle aches and tension 144, 165
muscular spasms 174
Mutual Arising of Liver/Lung Heat 134
Mycelized Children's Multiple Vitamins 77
myelitis 116
Myrobalan 112, 113
Myrrha 79, 80, 183, 269

Nagas 91
nasopharyngeal cavity 10

naturopathy 48, 138
Nei Jing 35, 36, 38, 45, 159, 163, 193, 265-266
Nei Ke 234
Nei Xie 164
Nei Yin 31
Neisseria Gonorrhoeae 10, 15
Neither Internal Nor External causes 31
Nelson *et al.* 8
neonatal infection 11
neoplasms 38, 61, 189
nephritis 254
nephrolithiasis 202
Neuro-linguistic Programming 92
New Flesh 72-76, 78, 183
New Medicine x, 153, 162
Nidus Vespae 183
Nine Ounces 53
NLP 92, 93
nocturia 196-197, 205, 209, 246-247
Nodulations 63, 65-67, 71, 72, 121, 199
non-smooth urination 238, 250
nosodes 96, 158, 160, 165, 210, 213, 227-228
Notopterygium 251
Nu Yin Kuei Yang 124
Nutmeg 113

O_2 137
obstruction when urinating 196
Obstructive Qi Stagnation 241, 250
OC use 15
OCs 12, 34, 100
Oleum Melaleucae Linariifoliae 74, 75
Oleum Semenis Lini Usitatissimi 225
Oleum Semenis Ricinis Communis 81
Oleum Sesami 74
Oleum Thujae Occidentalis 74, 75
Omphalia 112
On Prescription, Vol. 2 60
oncogenesis 189
oncogenic virus 11
Oncovin 6
Ootheca Mantidis 223
Opening the Pass Pills 236
oral, anal, and genital sex 10
oral cancer 116
oral contraceptives 12, 42, 99, 149
Orange Peel 146, 148, 149

Organic Germanium 85, 226
orgasm 93, 94, 204
orthomolecular therapy 78, 82-83, 89, 156, 158, 162, 212, 224, 253
Otsuka Keisetsu 118
Ou-yang Yi 236-238, 248, 250
Outer Kidneys 206
ovarian cancer 5
Oxy Toddy 132, 135, 137
ozone 137

Paget's disease 189
pain with intercourse 55
Painful Flow 30
pale tongue 48, 209, 240, 247
palpation 163, 196, 216-218, 229
palpitations 47, 62, 209, 238, 246
pancreas 107, 190
Pap smear viii, 2-3, 20-21, 27, 43, 94, 98, 162, 167-168, 187, 211
Papillon 83
papillomavirus 9
Papoviridae 14
papules 15, 19
paramesonephric ducts 191
paranasal sinuses 190
parasites 33, 76, 77, 100, 105, 108, 110, 122, 137
parasitosis 109, 110, 132, 138
parathyroid 190
paraxial mesoderm 190
Parkinson's disease 189
paroophoron 191
Parsley 135, 136
Parsley Root 136
Passion Flower 144
Pasta Ulmi Macrocarpi 111, 114
patency of Qi 31, 242, 250-251, 267
pathogenic bacteria 196
pathological vicariation 23
Pathways 29, 37, 265
Pattern (of Disharmony) 139, 140
Pau D'Arco 105, 137
Pauling, Dr. Linus 82
Pei Zheng-xue 154
pelvic exercise 54
penis 19, 21, 96, 172, 209
pentacyclic triterpenoids 275
pent-up Qi 56, 149
Peony 59, 69, 141, 143, 146-148, 174, 242, 245, 249
Peppermint 135, 136
peptidases 107
Periarteritis nodosa 189
Pericardium 216-218, 221
Pericarpium Arecae 250
Pericarpium Citri Reticulatae 63, 144, 148, 150, 240, 249
Pericarpium Citri Reticulatae Viride 63
Pericarpium Punicae Granati 110, 113
Pericarpium Viridis Citri Reticulatae 144, 149
perineal and low back pain 196
perineum 255
Periostracum Cicadae 181
periproctitis 177
peritonitis 177
persistent Heat 34, 37
persistent lesions 11
persistent, low-grade Heat 37
persistent viral infection 188, 276
Pestilential Qi 32
Phellodendron 104, 119, 247
Phellostatin 104
Phlegm 32, 53, 63, 66-67, 69-71, 75, 79, 84, 113, 118, 121, 123, 133, 144-150, 153-155, 166, 175, 216-217, 221
Phlegm Dampness Obstructing the Lungs 237
Phlegm Nodulation 118
Pi Fu Ke 171
PID 87
Pilates Method 55
Pinellia 69, 145, 146, 148, 176
Ping Wei San 150
Ping Xiao Dan 70, 123, 155, 219
Pizzorno & Murray 83, 156
Placenta Hominis 151
Plant & Contact Dermatitis 80
plantar warts 171
Platycodon 251
Pfeiffer, Carl C. 115
Plantain Leaf 133
plasters 72, 79, 80
Plastrum Testudinis 151
PMS 48, 58, 71, 87, 100, 101, 143, 144, 147, 148, 150, 158
pneumonia 116
Po 145
Polyporus 153

polyuria 6, 103, 209, 247, 254
Pomegranate 113
poor appetite 47, 154
porfiromycin 6
Poria 60, 69, 111, 143, 146, 148, 153, 222, 242, 244
Post Virotox 157, 227
Postnatal Kidney Yang 133
Postnatal production of Qi and Blood 130
Postnatal Qi 44, 239
postpartum lochia 32
Power Mushrooms 96, 152, 154, 214
prabhava 138
pre-TCM acupuncture 163
pregnancy 15, 17, 38, 40, 100
premenstrual breast and/or nipple pain 65
Premenstrual Breast Distention & Pain 58
premenstrual tension 149
premenstruum 74, 77, 80-82, 89, 99
Prenatal Qi 44
preventive treatment xii, 96, 129, 211
Principle of Similar Transformation 31, 41
Pritikin 53, 131, 271
Probioplex 106, 107
prodromal signs and symptoms 85, 117, 118, 196, 219
profuse leukorrhea 46, 48
Prostagen 224, 253
prostaglandin 275
prostate vii-xii, 61, 187-200, 201-202, 204-207, 210-213, 218-221, 223-225, 226-228, 233-234, 238-243, 251-255, 275-276
prostate cancer vii, 187, 189, 192-195, 197-202, 206-207, 210,211, 218-219, 227, 253
prostate capsule 199
prostatic calculi 198
Prostate Gland Pills 223
prostatic hypertrophy vii, 187-189, 195-197, 199-202, 209, 222, 234, 253, 275
prostatic specific antigen 198
prostatic tuberculosis 198
prostatic urethra
prostatic utricle 189, 191, 192
protease 107
protozoa 99, 228

Prunus Africana 275
PSA 198
PSCC 99-101, 103, 108
Pseudostellaria 144, 145
Psyllium Husks 135
Pueraria 142
Pulsatilla 104
Pulvis Corticis Phellodendri 73
Pulvis Floris Carthami 80
Pulvis Fructi Crataegi 80
Pulvis Herbae Larreae 73
Pulvis Indigo Naturalis 66
Pulvis Radicis Achyranthis 80
Pulvis Radicis Lithospermi Seu Arnebiae 73
Pulvis Radicis Paeoniae Albae 80
Pulvis Radicis Salviae Miltorrhizae 80
Pulvis Radicis Saussureae Seu Vladimiriae 80
Pumpkin Seeds 225
punch biopsy 2
punch suprapubic cystostomy 199
Pure of the Impure of Liquids and Foods 102
pus in the urine 198
Pygeum Africanum 275-276
Pyridoxine 13
pyuria 198

Qi and Blood Deficiency 61
Qi Congestion 34, 41, 140, 146, 203
Qi Dribbling 203
Qi Fen 36
Qi Gong 55, 212
Qi Hai 55, 102, 192
Qi Hai/Dan Tian 55
Qi Jing Ba Mai 163, 229
Qi Lin 201, 203, 229, 250
Qi Men 44
Qi Stagnation/Liver Depression 47
Qi Wu Jiang Xia Tang 118
Qian Lie Xian Wan 202, 223, 253
Qian Ri Chuang 171
Qing Fei Yi Huo Wan 235
Qing or purplish tongue 54
Qing Peng San 73
Qing Re, Jie Du 65
Qing Xin Lian Zi Yin 238-239
Qing Xue 68, 75
Qu Gu 228

Qu Mai Tang 250
Qu Quan 126
Qu Xie 64, 74, 76, 78, 105
Qualiherbs 62, 118, 141-142, 174, 178, 180, 214, 252, 277
Quell Fire 124
Quisqualis 110, 112

radical hysterectomy 5, 6
radical prostatectomy 200
radiculitis 116
radiotherapy 6
Radix Achyranthis 223
Radix Altheae Officinalis 269
Radix Angelicae Sinensis 59, 60, 62-63, 74, 119, 125-126, 142-143, 146, 174, 179-183, 240, 242, 249-250
Radix Asteris 238
Radix Astragali Seu Hedysari 62, 117, 119, 179, 223, 239
Radix Bupleuri 59, 60, 63, 69, 117, 124, 125, 150, 240
Radix Chelidonii Majus 182
Radix Codonopsis Pilosulae 104, 110, 117, 126, 223
Radix Collinsoniae Canadensis 220-221
Radix Dioscoreae 247-248
Radix Dioscoreae Oppositae 104, 117
Radix Euphorbiae Kansui 252
Radix Et Rhizoma Gentianae Campestris 120
Radix Fraserae Carolinensis 120
Radix Glehniae 238
Radix Gentianae Scabrae 124, 125
Radix Glycyrrhizae 104, 111, 117, 124, 125, 150, 174, 175, 177-179, 181, 183, 223, 237, 239-240, 242-243, 249
Radix Helionadis Dioicae 220, 221
Radix Hydrangeae Arborscentis 230
Radix Hydrocotylis Asiaticae 143, 144
Radix Isatidis 68, 117
Radix Ledebouriellae Sesloides 181
Radix Ligustici Chuanxiong 63, 119, 141, 178-180
Radix Lithospermi Seu Arnebiae 68, 179, 182, 183
Radix Lindera 249
Radix Paeoniae Albae 59, 60, 63, 69, 119, 143, 146, 174, 179-180, 242, 249
Radix Paeoniae Albae Seu Rubrae 63
Radix Panacis Ginseng Seu Codonopsis Pilosulae 62, 69
Radix Patriniae Heterophyllae 64, 65
Radix Petroselini 136
Radix Peucidani 223, 235
Radix Platycodi 235, 250
Radix Polygalae Tenuifoliae 62
Radix Praeparatus Aconiti Carmichaeli 176, 248
Radix Praeparatus Glycyrrhizae 59-60, 62, 69, 144, 148, 249
Radix Pseudostellariae Heterophyllae 143, 144
Radix Puerariae 142
Radix Rehmanniae 63, 68, 119, 124-125, 180-181, 223, 239, 246-248
Radix Rubiae Cordifoliae 110, 113
Radix Rumicis 133, 134
Radix Salviae Miltorrhizae 63, 223, 252
Radix Scrophulariae 68
Radix Scutellariae Baicalensis 124, 125, 143, 145, 177, 180, 235, 239, 243
Radix Scutellariae Barbatae 63
Radix Sophorae Flavescentis 67, 125, 181, 235
Radix Symphyti Officinalis 74, 75, 183
Radix Trichosanthis Kirlowii 144, 147, 235
Rambling Powder 59
Ramulus Cinnamomi 69, 174, 240, 244, 252
rapid eye movements 230
rapidly progressive poorly differentiated squamous carcinomas 22
Raw Prostate Concentrate 224, 225
Re Lin 145, 153, 201, 222
Realgar powder 126, 237
Rebellious Qi 121, 145, 150
recreational drugs 39, 212
rectal digital exam 187
rectal mucosa 110
rectum 6, 89, 198, 262
recurrent condyloma 18
recurrent stomatitis 116
Red Clover 134
Red Dates 69, 142, 147, 148
regressive vicariation 23
regulation of the hormones 59
Rehmannia 6 Flavor Pills 246
Rehmannia 8 Flavor Pills 248

311

Reichian body-typing 216, 218
Reid, Richard 1
reinfection 17, 94, 95, 169
relapsing urinary tract infections 196
Relaxed Wanderer 141
REM 230
remedial exercise 53-56
remedial treatment viii, 51, 54, 93, 96, 99, 129-130, 223, 233, 234
Removing Firewood Brew 243
renal failure 197
repeat Pap 21, 22, 59, 98, 167, 270
Repletion 31
Resina Rhi Verniciferae 67
resonance filters 96, 101, 129, 157, 210, 227-228
respiratory tract 190, 225
restlessness 144, 148
retroviruses 188
Return the Spleen Decoction 61
Return to Nest 88
rheumatic problems 714
rheumatoid arthritis 189
Rhizoma Acori Graminei 249, 252
Rhizoma Alismatis 124, 126, 223, 237, 240, 243, 244, 247, 248
Rhizoma Arisaematis 67
Rhizoma Atractylodis 59, 60, 62, 63, 104, 110, 117, 118, 142, 150, 174, 178, 181, 240, 252
Rhizoma Atractylodis Macrocephalae 59, 60, 62, 63, 110, 142, 150, 240, 252
Rhizoma Belamcandae Chinensis 250
Rhizoma Cimicifugae 179, 240
Rhizoma Coptidis 125, 177, 180, 250
Rhizoma Corydalis Yanhusuo 250
Rhizoma Cyperi 126, 141, 144, 147
Rhizoma Cyperi Rotundae 141
Rhizoma Dioscoreae Hypoglaucae 220, 222, 243, 249, 252
Rhizoma Drynariae 182
Rhizoma Et Radix Notopterygii 250
Rhizoma Gusuibu 182
Rhizoma Hydrastis Canadensis 120
Rhizoma Imperatae 236
Rhizoma Paridis Polyphyllae 64
Rhizoma Pinelliae Ternatae 69, 143, 145, 150, 177, 237
Rhizoma Polygonati Officinalis 238
Rhizoma Recens Zingiberis 59, 62, 69, 110, 150, 240
Rhizoma Rhei 134, 178, 179, 235, 242, 245, 250
Rhizoma Sanguinariae Canadensis 120, 121
Rhizoma Smilacis Glabrae 66, 126, 178
Rhizoma Zedoariae 67
Rhubarb 178, 245
Richart, Ralph M. 1, 18
Righteous Fire of Middle and Lower Burners 133, 206
Righteous Qi 23, 44, 127, 213, 215, 217, 219
Riley, David, MD 159
risk factors in genital HPV infection 15
RNA 8, 10, 20
Root disharmony 70
Root treatments 89
roundworms 112
rubella 169, 188
rubeola 169, 188
Rubia 113

sacral ganglia 116
sadhanas 91
sadness and depression 103
Sal Nitri 70, 71
Salmonella Dublin 107
Salvia 63, 227, 252
San Bao 44
San Yin Jiao 90, 126
Sandy *Lin* 202
Sanguinaria 121
saprophyte 99
sarcodes 158
sarcoma of the prostate 198
Saussurea 111, 150
Saussurea Regulate the Qi Pills 150
Saw Palmetto Berries 220-221, 225
Scanty Menstrual Flow 97
Scatter Wind Powder 180
schizophrenia 189
School of Attack & Purgation 155
Schussler cell salts 158
sciatica 43
Scientific Botanicals 83, 277
Sclerotium Polypori Umbellati 152, 235, 237. 240
Sclerotium Poriae Cocoris 42, 59-60, 62-63, 69, 110, 178 142-143, 146, 152,

220, 237, 239-240, 242, 244, 247-249, 252
Scutellaria 63, 69, 145, 235
Scutellaria & Gardenia Combination 235
Scutellaria Clear the Lungs Drink 235
Sea of Blood 192
Sea Seal 254
Seem, Mark 163
Selenium 13, 83, 84, 224, 226, 253
Semen Abutilonis Seu Malvae 220, 222, 249, 252
Semen Arecae Catechu 110, 112, 237
Semen Benincasae Hispidae 178, 245
Semen Cannabis 226
Semen Coicis Lachryma-jobi 173-176, 179, 244
Semen Cuscutae 223, 248
Semen Nelumbinis 239
Semen Pharbitidis 250
Semen Phaseoli Calcarati 235, 236
Semen Plantaginis 104, 124, 223, 239, 242, 248, 252
Semen Pruni Armeniacae 175, 237
Semen Pruni Persicae 178, 244, 245
Semen Sesami Indici 181
Semen Strychnotis 67, 70, 71
Semen Torreyae Grandis 110
Semen Vaccariae Segetalis 223, 249, 252
Semen Zizyphi Spinosae 62
senile insomnia 206
septum transverum 190
sessile papules 15, 19
Seven Forests 142, 150, 277
Seven Passions 31, 32
severe dysplasia 1-5, 13, 74, 85
sex during menstruation 32, 93, 166, 167
sexual fatigue 203
sexual pacing 212, 231-232
sexually transmitted disease 7, 194
sexually transmitted Evil Qi 179
Sha Jun 77, 100, 109, 113, 123
Sha Lin 202
shamanic medicine 91
Shan Bing 118, 254
Shang Han Lun 142, 161
Shanghai College of TCM 164
Shao Fu Tong 30, 87, 175, 176

Shao Shang 164, 165
Shao Yang 121, 133, 145, 149, 217
Shao Yang Fen 121, 133
Shao Yin 218
Shaolin Patriarch De Chan 145
Shen 44, 56, 60-61, 68, 80, 84, 103, 108, 145, 147, 150, 166, 206, 242-243, 248, 264
Shen Nong Ben Cao Jing 147
Shen Qi Wan 248
Shen Qu 108
Shen Que 80
Shen Spirit 103
Sheng Hua 102, 119, 208, 241
Shi Er Zheng Jing 163
Shi Lin 201, 222
Shiitake 152, 153
shortness of breath 47, 236
Shui Dao 234
Shui Niu Jiao 68
Shui Zhen 82, 227-228
Shui Zhong 222
Si Fen 36
Si Ni 54
Si Wu Tang 63, 119
Si Yao Yo Gao 74
Similia similibus currantur 159
Simonton, O. Carl 92
sinovial membranes 190
sinu-utricular cord 191
sitz baths 255
Sivin, Nathan 45
Six *Fen* 36
Six Great Medicines 114
Six Stagnations 32, 123, 229
Sixbey *et al.* 11
skin cancer 10, 67
skin irritation 80
skin rashes 165
SLE 93, 189
Slippery Elm suppositories 270
small intestine 6, 67, 103, 107, 209, 216-218, 225, 234, 238
smegma 10
Smilax 126, 178
smoking 12, 33, 34, 40, 52
Soaring Dragon Decoction 177, 178
Solaray 276, 277
sore throat 47
Sou Shuo 202

313

Southern blot test 20
Sp 10 126
Sp 15 217
Sp 6 90, 126
Sp 9 126
spermatorrhea 134
spermatozoa 10
Spina Gleditschiae 237
Spirit 44, 60, 84, 91, 103, 113, 138, 146, 148, 152-154, 158, 161, 163, 218, 224, 265
Spleen 47-48, 52, 59-61, 65-70, 75, 84, 100, 103-105, 106-112, 114, 118, 121-122, 126, 140-141, 143-150, 152-154, 157, 173-174, 203, 208-209, 216-218, 221, 226-227, 239, 241, 254-266
Spleen Dampness 109, 148, 150, 174, 217
Spleen Earth 60
Spleen Qi Deficiency 47, 48, 61, 109, 140
Spleen/Small Intestine Deficiency 209
Spleen *Yun Hua* function 108
Spleen/Blood Activator 157
Spleen/Kidney Dual Deficiency 47
spotting after coitus 30
Spring Pond Decoction 240
squamous cell carcinoma of prostate 198
squamous metaplasia 15
St. 25 216
St 29 80
Stage A-D 199
Stagnant Blood 6, 32, 40-42, 48, 63-67, 75, 79, 80, 88, 98, 113, 134, 141, 142, 155, 178, 179, 183, 202, 204, 206, 216, 221, 245, 249, 251252
Stagnant Blood in the Lower Burner 48, 178, 179, 245
Stagnant Dampness 41, 217
Stagnant Food 41, 108, 216
Stagnant Qi and Blood with Mutual Entanglement of   Damp Heat 30
Stagnant Toxins 46
Stagnation and Accumulation 76, 81, 98, 105, 183, 250
Stagnation Dispelling Pill 123
Stagnation in the *Luo* 71
Stagnation of Damp Heat in the Lower Burner 61

Stagnation of Qi 31-32, 35, 54, 147, 154, 205, 231
Stagnation of Qi and Blood 31, 35, 54, 147, 205, 231
STD 7, 8, 15, 21, 33, 37, 95, 178, 179, 194, 195
sterols 275-276
steroids 99
Stoff and Pelegrino, Drs. 276
Stomach 36, 53, 60, 65-70, 75, 84, 102-103, 105-107, 108, 111, 121-122, 126, 130, 134-136, 145-150, 153-154, 180, 209, 216-218, 222, 226, 235, 239
stomach acid 135
Stomach Fluids 60
Stomach Heat 60, 209, 216
Stomach/Lung/Liver Heat 147
Stone *Lin* 201
Stone Root 221
stress 39, 41, 48, 52, 56, 82, 99, 143, 149, 184, 194, 204, 208, 238, 250, 276
striae 80, 266
Stuck Qi 31, 34
stuffy chest 237
subclinical condyloma 18
subclinical genital HPV infections 18
Sui Marrow 164
suis organ preparations 158
Sun Si-miao 231
Superficial Wind Invasion 236
suppositories 72, 73, 76-78, 270
Surface 1, 6, 24, 44, 88, 102-103, 115-116, 121, 146, 164-165, 174-175, 225
surface erythema 6
surgical castration 200
surgical erosion 25
surgical excision 182
Swertia Chirata 120
swollen tongue 30
syphilis 15, 37, 195
syphlitic bubo 178
syphlitis keratitis 178
syphlitis skin lesion 178
Szechuan Pepper 114

T4/T8 cell ratio 17
T cell count 43
Taheebo 105
Tai Du 194
Tai Ji 55, 212, 230

Tai Qi Chuan 213
Tai Lou 38
Tai Ping Hui Min He Ji Chu Fang 140
Tai Yang 217, 234
Tai Yin 217
Taiwanese empirical formula for treatment of cervical cancer 62
Talc 235, 242, 244, 249, 252
tampon 72, 76-78, 156, 269
Tang Dynasty 160, 231
Tang Kuei & Gambir Combination 118, 214
Tangerine Peel 149
Tantric Buddhism 91
TCM *Bian Zheng* diagnosis 27, 100, 151, 234
TCM *Bian Zheng* of cervical cancer 46
TCM descriptions of cervical cancer 28
TCM functional definition 44
TCM gynecology 29, 72
TCM methodology 27, 31, 57
Tea Tree Oil 75, 76, 182, 269
Teng Long Tang 177, 245
temperamental Organ 31
terminal dribbling 197, 233, 252
testitis 177
testosterone 192, 193, 200, 206-207, 219
TH 1 164
Thallus Algae 117, 118
The Golden Mirror of the Medical Tradition 101
The Healing Nutrients Within 115
The New England Journal of Medicine 188
The Yeast Syndrome 101, 104
thirst 112, 147, 235, 238
Thlaspi 175, 176
Thorny Condition 171
Thousand Day Lesions 171
Three Burners 37, 104, 119, 234
Three Free Therapies 57, 89, 99, 129, 162
Three Treasures 44
Three Wrathful Lords 91
thrush 108
Thuja 75, 76, 159, 182, 269
Thuja Occidentalis 159,
Thuja Oil 75, 76, 182, 269
thymus 190

thyroid 65, 190
thyroid cancers 65
Ti Gang Ji 127
Tian Shu 216
Tiao Jing Gao 79, 80
Tibetan medical theory 110, 166
Tic douloureux 116
Tierra, Michael 144
tinnitus 47, 209, 246
tobacco 11, 34
Tokoro 222, 243, 248, 251
Tokoro Separate the Clear Drink 248, 251
Tong Guan Wan 236
Tong Jing 30, 58, 80, 86, 97, 176
topical treatment of warts 181
Torreya 112
total hysterectomy 5
Townsend, Duane E. 21
Toxins 35, 39, 46, 48-49, 63-67, 72, 74-77, 79, 84-85, 99, 100, 105, 107, 118, 120-122, 125-126, 133-134, 137, 144, 147, 157-158, 160, 164, 172, 180, 182-183, 194, 205, 214, 220, 226, 253
tracheobronchitis 116
Traditional Chinese Medicine vii, 26, 28, 29, 36, 68, 167, 168, 191, 193, 236
trans-activation of the HPV genome 11
transmission from Inside to Outside 164
transrectal ultrasound 198
transurethral resection 199
traumatic herpes 116
traumatic injury 113, 133, 204
Treating Cancer with Chinese Herbs 62
treatment of sexual partners 95
Treponema Pallidum 10, 15
Trichloracetic Acid 22
Trichomonas Vaginalis 10, 15
Trichosanthes 147, 148
trigeminal neuralgia 43, 116
trigone 190
Triple Heater 45, 102, 132, 138, 147, 165, 216-218, 225, 234, 264, 266
Tuber Curcumae 70
tumor 6, 8, 88, 105, 261, 275
Tung Ching-chang 254
Turbid *Lin* 202
Turbid Urinary Disturbance 153

315

Turbidity 104-105, 110-111, 183, 216, 248
Two Aged Decoction with Additions 237
Two Yin 76, 79
typhoid 35
typhus 35

Ulceration of the Female Genitalia 124
ulcerations of the skin 6
ulcers, small 238
Ulmus 114
Ultrabifidus 106, 107
Ultradophilus 77, 106, 107, 156
ultramolecular 157, 159
unaided visible detection 19
unconventional viruses 188
undifferentiated prostatic carcinoma 198
unprotected sex 94, 210-211, 213, 232
Unschuld, Paul U. 45
Upper Burner 36, 61, 69, 145, 234, 247
uremia 197
urethra 20, 76, 96, 189-191, 197, 208
urethral catheterization 199
urinary frequency and urgency 196
urinary gravel 202
urinary retention 197, 199, 201
urinary tract infection 196, 197
urination 66-67, 69, 112, 133-134, 136, 146, 153, 173, 197, 202-203, 205, 208-209, 220, 222, 225-226, 233, 235, 238, 240-242, 246, 248-250, 252
urine 20, 46, 197-198, 208-209, 233, 236, 241, 246, 259
urogenital sinus 191
urogenital system 190
Uterine Qi and Blood Stagnation 167
uterine tumors 178
Uterus 5, 34, 36, 88, 145, 191
UTI 197

vaccinations 160
vaginal and anal pruritus 100
Vaginal Depletion Packs 76
vaginal douches 78
vaginal infection 58
Vaginal Lesions 58, 127
vaginal meatus 127
vaginal syringe 78, 79

Vajrapani 91
varicella 169
Vega biokinesiology 156, 157, 210, 213, 227
Vegatesting 96, 157, 213, 227
venereal diseases 8, 36, 37, 118, 178, 195
venereal *Fu Xie* 38
venereal transmission 10, 11, 15, 195, 202
verrucae 172, 173, 176
vesicular skin eruptions 116
vestigial duct 191
VIN 24, 25
vincristine 6
vinegar 19, 80, 96, 106, 269, 272
viral infection ix, 8, 12, 72, 115, 171, 180, 188, 202-203, 210, 213-215, 219, 226, 276
viral proteins 8, 10
viral replication/particles 14
ViraPap 20, 129, 168, 209-210, 213
virus specific RNA 10
Vis Mediatrix Naturae 92, 93
visualization 90-92
Vitamin A 13, 75, 78, 269-270
Vitamin C 13, 83, 84, 226, 253
Vitamin E 83, 84, 225
vitamin/mineral deficiencies 12
vitamins 77, 82-83, 85, 137, 156-157, 228
vomiting 121, 238
vulva 19, 22, 23
vulvar condylomata 22, 24
vulvar intraepithelial neoplasia 24
vulvectomy 25
vulvovaginitis 116

Wai Ke 49, 171
Wai Yin 31-33, 77
Wai Shen 206
Warm Disease theory ix, 35
Warm Evil 35, 36, 39, 117, 129, 194, 207, 209
Warm Evil Disease 35
Warm External Evil 36
Warm Hidden Evils 37, 38
Warm the Essence Drink 179
Water Buffalo Horn 68
Water Needle therapy 82, 227

Water Passageways 234, 236
Wei Fen 36, 37
Wei Qi 32, 34-45, 102, 164-165, 174, 180, 212, 221, 266
Wei Tong 139
Wen Bing ix, 33, 35, 36, 38, 164
Wen Fa 127
Wen Fu Xie Qi 37, 39
Wen Hua 249
Wen Jing Yin 179
Wen Re 37, 54, 183
Wen Xie 37, 42, 67-68, 117, 127, 154, 164-165, 172, 179, 194, 197, 202, 205, 210, 212, 229
Wen Yi Lun 32
Western epidemiology 36
Western etiologies of cervical dysplasia 7, 33
Western immune system 43, 45
White Cloud 88
White Tree Ear 153
Wind Evil 172
Wind Heat Invasion 236
Wiseman and Ellis 67
Wolfe, Honora Lee 53
Wooden Woman 87
worm 33, 112
Wu Dai 29
Wu Ju-tong 35, 37
Wu Lin 201-202, 241
Wu Lin San 241
Wu Pi San 152
Wu Qian 101
Wu Shu Xue 229
Wu Wei 139
Wu You-ke 32
Wu Yun Liu Qi 32
Wu Zi Wan 152

Xia Yi Xue 90
Xiang Chuan Jie Du Ji 178
Xiao Feng San 180
Xiao Yao San 59-64, 85, 140-142
Xie Qi 37, 39, 44, 48, 91, 172
Xin Yi 153, 154
Xing Jian 126
Xu Li 68
Xue Fen 36, 37, 67, 68, 115, 165, 180, 183, 194
Xue Hai 126, 192

Xue Lin 201, 222
Xue Zheng Lun Ping Shi 154

Yan Yun Liao Fa 127
Yang Excess 206, 215-219
Yang Fire 165, 206-207
Yang Ming 107, 149
Yang Qi 93, 146, 265-267
Ye Tian-shi 35
yeast 33, 77, 99-101, 103-106, 108-110, 114, 138, 228, 272-273
yeast-free diet 106
Yellow Bell 34
Yellow Discharge 29
Yellow Dock 134
Yerba Prima Botanicals 132, 277
Yerba Prima Internal Cleansing Program 132
Yi Yi Fu Zi Bai Jiang San 175
Yi Yi Ren Tang 174, 175
Yi Xue Xin Wu 252
Yi Zong Jin Jian 101
Yin Accumulation 174, 184
Yin Chuang 58
Yin Deficiency insomnia 154
Yin Essence 206
Yin Excess 215-217
Yin Gu 126
Yin Healing Powder 72, 73
Yin *Jing* tonics 151
Yin Ling Quan 126
Ying 36, 37, 148, 266
Ying Fen 36
Yong Yang 175, 177
Yoo Tae-woo 215, 229
Yu Men Jiang 127
Yuan 35, 44, 45, 155, 185, 248
Yuan Original Qi 44, 45, 185
Yuan Source Qi 44
Yue Jing Guo Duo 64, 97
Yue Jing Guo Shao 97
Yue Qu Wan 123
Yun 32, 44, 88, 108, 127, 155
Yun Bai 88

Zang Fu 45, 69, 103, 149, 164, 219, 263
Zanthoxylum 114
zenomolecular 156, 157, 159, 160, 162
Zhang Jing-yue 191
Zhang Zi-he 155

317

Zhen Qi 44
Zheng Jia Ji Ju 81
Zheng Qi 37, 44-46, 82, 126, 136, 164, 180, 184-185, 217
Zhi Bai Di Huang Wan 247
Zhu Dan-xi 248
Zhu Xue 87
Zhuo Lin 153, 202, 207, 229
Zi Cao Gao 182, 183
Zi Gen Mu Li Tang 179
Zi Gong Kou 192
Zi Gong Xue 80
Zinc 13, 83, 84, 156, 253
Zinc and Copper needles 229
Zong 34, 101, 192
Zur Hausen and Fenoglio 10

OTHER BOOKS ON CHINESE MEDICINE AVAILABLE FROM BLUE POPPY PRESS

1775 Linden Ave
Boulder, CO 80304
303\442-0796

SECOND SPRING: A Guide To Healthy Menopause Through Traditional Chinese Medicine by Honora Lee Wolfe ISBN 0-936185-18-X $12.95

STICKING TO THE POINT: A Rational Methodology for the Step by Step Formulation & Administration of an Acupuncture Treatment by Bob Flaws ISBN 0-936185-17-1 $14.95

MIGRAINES & TRADITIONAL CHINESE MEDICINE: A Layperson's Guide by Bob Flaws ISBN 0-936185-15-5 $11.95

ENDOMETRIOSIS & INFERTILITY AND TRADITIONAL CHINESE MEDICINE: A Laywoman's Guide by Bob Flaws ISBN 0-936185-14-7 $9.95

CLASSICAL MOXIBUSTION SKILLS IN CONTEMPORARY CLINICAL PRACTICE by Sung Baek ISBN 0-936185-16-3 $10.95

THE BREAST CONNECTION: A Laywoman's Guide to the Treatment of Breast Disease by Chinese Medicine by Honora Lee Wolfe ISBN 0-936185-13-9 $8.95

NINE OUNCES: A Nine Part Program For The Prevention of AIDS in HIV Positive Persons by Bob Flaws ISBN 0-936185-12-0 $8.95

THE TREATMENT OF CANCER BY INTEGRATED CHINESE-WESTERN MEDICINE by Zhang Dai-zhao, trans. by Zhang Ting-liang & Bob Flaws, ISBN 0-936185-11-2 $16.95

BLUE POPPY ESSAYS: 1988 Translations and Ruminations on Chinese Medicine by Bob Flaws, et al, ISBN 0-936185-10-4 $18.95

A HANDBOOK OF TRADITIONAL CHINESE DERMATOLOGY by

Liang Jian-hui, trans. by Zhang Ting-liang & Bob Flaws, ISBN 0-936185-07-4 $14.95

SECRET SHAOLIN FORMULAE FOR THE TREATMENT OF EXTERNAL INJURY by Patriarch De Chan, trans. by Zhang Ting-liang & Bob Flaws, ISBN 0-936185-08-2 $12.95

A HANDBOOK OF TRADITIONAL CHINESE GYNECOLOGY by Zhejiang College of TCM, trans. by Zhang Ting-liang, ISBN 0-936185-06-6 $17.95

FREE & EASY: Traditional Chinese Gynecology for American Women 2nd Edition, by Bob Flaws, ISBN 0-936185-05-8 $15.95

PRINCE WEN HUI'S COOK: Chinese Dietary Therapy by Bob Flaws & Honora Lee Wolfe, ISBN 0-912111-05-4, $12.95 (Published by Paradigm Press, Brookline, MA)

TURTLE TAIL & OTHER TENDER MERCIES: Traditional Chinese Pediatrics by Bob Flaws ISBN 0-936185-00-7 $14.95

ABOUT THE AUTHOR

Bob Flaws, DOM, CMT, Dipl.Ac., is an internationally known practitioner of and author on traditional Chinese medicine. He has written, translated, and edited over a dozen books on various aspects of Oriental medicine. Numerous articles by Dr. Flaws have appeared in professional journals both in America and abroad. In addition, Dr. Flaws regularly lectures at many of the major American colleges of acupuncture and Oriental medicine and has been an invited speaker at many national and international medical conferences.

Dr. Flaws originally studied acupuncture with Dr. Tao Xi-yu. He also studied acupuncture, Chinese herbal medicine, and Tuina massage at the Shanghai College of Traditional Chinese Medicine. He is a founding member and past member of the Board of Directors of the Acupuncture Association of Colorado, a member of the American Association of Acupuncture and Oriental Medicine, was appointed a Research Associate of the Tibetan Medical Society, and is a graduate of the Boulder School of Massage Therapy.